The Princeton Review®

MCAT®

General Chemistry Review, 3rd Edition

The Staff of The Princeton Review

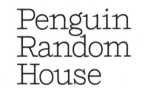

Penguin
Random
House

The Princeton Review

The Princeton Review
24 Prime Parkway, Suite 201
Natick, MA 01760
E-mail: editorialsupport@review.com

Published in the United States by Penguin Random House LLC, New York, and in Canada by Random House of Canada, a division of Penguin Random House Ltd., Toronto.

ISBN: 978-1-101-92057-2
ISSN: 2150-8879

MCAT is a registered trademark of the Association of American Medical Colleges, which does not sponsor or endorse this product.

The Princeton Review is not affiliated with Princeton University.

Editor: Aaron Riccio
Production Artist: Deborah A. Silvestrini
Production Editors: Beth Hanson, Kiley Pulliam,
                      Harmony Quiroz

Printed in the United States of America on partially recycled paper.

10 9 8 7 6

3rd Edition

Editorial

Rob Franek, Senior VP, Publisher
Casey Cornelius, VP Content Development
Mary Beth Garrick, Director of Production
Selena Coppock, Managing Editor
Meave Shelton, Senior Editor
Colleen Day, Editor
Sarah Litt, Editor
Aaron Riccio, Editor
Orion McBean, Editorial Assistant

Random House Publishing Team

Tom Russell, Publisher
Alison Stoltzfus, Publishing Manager
Melinda Ackell, Associate Managing Editor
Ellen Reed, Production Manager
Kristin Lindner, Production Supervisor
Andrea Lau, Designer

CONTRIBUTORS

Steven A. Leduc
    Senior Author
Kendra Bowman
    Ph.D., Senior Author

TPR MCAT G-Chem Development Team:
Bethany Blackwell, M.S., William Ewing, Ph.D., Chris Fortenbach, B.S.

Senior Editor, Lead Developer
Bethany Blackwell, M.S.

Edited for Production by:
Judene Wright, M.S., M.A.Ed.
    National Content Director, MCAT Program, The Princeton Review

The TPR MCAT G-Chem Team and Judene would like to thank the following people for their contributions to this book :

Patrick Abulencia, Ph.D., Kashif Anwar, M.D., M.M.S., Argun Can, Brian Cato, Nita Chauhan, H.BSc, MSc, Rob Fong, M.D., Ph.D., Neil Maluste, B.S., Chris Manuel, M.P.H., Douglas K. McLemore, B.S., Marion-Vincent L. Mempin, B.S., Donna Memran, Brian Mikolasko, M.D., M.BA, Katherine Miller, Ph. D., Steven Rines, Ph.D., Andrew Snyder, Danish Vaiyani, Christopher Volpe, Ph.D.

Periodic Table of the Elements

1 H 1.0																	2 He 4.0
3 Li 6.9	4 Be 9.0											5 B 10.8	6 C 12.0	7 N 14.0	8 O 16.0	9 F 19.0	10 Ne 20.2
11 Na 23.0	12 Mg 24.3											13 Al 27.0	14 Si 28.1	15 P 31.0	16 S 32.1	17 Cl 35.5	18 Ar 39.9
19 K 39.1	20 Ca 40.1	21 Sc 45.0	22 Ti 47.9	23 V 50.9	24 Cr 52.0	25 Mn 54.9	26 Fe 55.8	27 Co 58.9	28 Ni 58.7	29 Cu 63.5	30 Zn 65.4	31 Ga 69.7	32 Ge 72.6	33 As 74.9	34 Se 79.0	35 Br 79.9	36 Kr 83.8
37 Rb 85.5	38 Sr 87.6	39 Y 88.9	40 Zr 91.2	41 Nb 92.9	42 Mo 95.9	43 Tc (98)	44 Ru 101.1	45 Rh 102.9	46 Pd 106.4	47 Ag 107.9	48 Cd 112.4	49 In 114.8	50 Sn 118.7	51 Sb 121.8	52 Te 127.6	53 I 126.9	54 Xe 131.9
55 Cs 132.9	56 Ba 137.3	57 *La 138.9	72 Hf 178.5	73 Ta 180.9	74 W 183.9	75 Re 186.2	76 Os 190.2	77 Ir 192.2	78 Pt 195.1	79 Au 197.0	80 Hg 200.6	81 Tl 204.4	82 Pb 207.2	83 Bi 209.0	84 Po (209)	85 At (210)	86 Rn (222)
87 Fr (223)	88 Ra 226.0	89 †Ac 227.0	104 Rf (261)	105 Db (262)	106 Sg (266)	107 Bh (264)	108 Hs (277)	109 Mt (268)	110 Ds (281)	111 Rg (272)	112 Cn (285)	113 Uut (286)	114 Fl (289)	115 Uup (288)	116 Lv (293)	117 Uus (294)	118 Uuo (294)

*Lanthanide Series:

58 Ce 140.1	59 Pr 140.9	60 Nd 144.2	61 Pm (145)	62 Sm 150.4	63 Eu 152.0	64 Gd 157.3	65 Tb 158.9	66 Dy 162.5	67 Ho 164.9	68 Er 167.3	69 Tm 168.9	70 Yb 173.0	71 Lu 175.0

†Actinide Series:

90 Th 232.0	91 Pa (231)	92 U 238.0	93 Np (237)	94 Pu (244)	95 Am (243)	96 Cm (247)	97 Bk (247)	98 Cf (251)	99 Es (252)	100 Fm (257)	101 Md (258)	102 No (259)	103 Lr (260)

MCAT GENERAL CHEMISTRY CONTENTS

CONTENTS

MCAT MATH FOR GENERAL CHEMISTRY

Register Your

1 Go to **PrincetonReview.com/cracking**

2 You'll see a welcome page where you should register your book or boxed set of books using the ISBN. If you have a book, the ISBN can be found above the bar code on the back cover. If you have a boxed set, the ISBN can be found on the back of the box above the bar code.

3 After placing this free order, you'll either be asked to log in or to answer a few simple questions in order to set up a new Princeton Review account.

4 Finally, click on the "Student Tools" tab located at the top of the screen. It may take an hour or two for your registration to go through, but after that, you're good to go.

NOTE: If you are experiencing book problems (potential content errors), please contact EditorialSupport@review.com with the full title of the book, its ISBN number, and the page number of the error.

Experiencing technical issues? Please email TPRStudentTech@review.com with the following information:

· your full name

· e-mail address used to register the book

· full book title and ISBN

· your computer OS (Mac or PC) and Internet browser (Firefox, Safari, Chrome, etc.)

· description of technical issue

Book Online!

Once you've registered, you can...

- Take 3 full-length practice MCAT exams
- Find useful information about taking the MCAT and applying to medical school
- Check to see if there have been any updates to this edition

Offline Resources

If you are looking for more review or medical school advice, please feel free to pick up these books in stores right now!

- *Medical School Essays That Made a Difference*
- *The Best 167 Medical Schools*
- *The Princeton Review Complete MCAT*

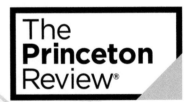

Chapter 7
Phases

7.1 PHYSICAL CHANGES

Matter can undergo physical changes as well as chemical changes. Melting, freezing, and boiling are all examples of physical changes. A key property of a physical change is that no *intra*molecular bonds are made or broken; a physical change affects only the *inter*molecular forces between molecules or atoms. For example, ice melting to become liquid water does not change the molecules of H_2O into something else. Melting reflects the disruption of the attractive interactions between the molecules.

Every type of matter experiences intermolecular forces such as dispersion forces, dipole interactions, and hydrogen bonding. All molecules have some degree of attraction towards each other (dispersion forces at least), and it's the intermolecular interactions that hold matter together as solids or liquids. The strength and the type of intermolecular forces depend on the identity of the atoms and molecules of a substance and vary greatly. For example, $NaCl(s)$, $H_2O(l)$ and $N_2(g)$ all have different kinds and strengths of intermolecular forces, and these differences give rise to their widely varying melting and boiling points.

Phase Transitions

Physical changes are closely related to temperature. What does temperature tell us about matter? Temperature is a measure of the amount of internal kinetic energy (the energy of motion) that molecules have. The average kinetic energy of the molecules of a substance directly affects its **state** or **phase**: whether it's a **solid**, **liquid**, or **gas**. Kinetic energy is also related to the degree of disorder, or **entropy**. In general, the higher the average kinetic energy of the molecules of a substance, the greater its entropy.

solid   liquid   gas

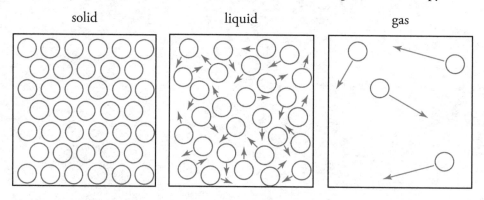

If we increase the temperature at a given pressure, a solid typically transforms into liquid and then into gas. What causes the phase transitions as the temperature increases? Phase changes are simply the result of breaking (or forming) intermolecular interactions. At low temperatures, matter tends to exist as a solid and is held together by intermolecular interactions. The molecules in a solid may jiggle a bit, but they're restricted to relatively fixed positions and form an orderly array, because the molecules don't have enough kinetic energy to overcome the intermolecular forces. Solids are the most ordered and least energetic of the phases. As a solid absorbs heat its temperature increases, meaning the average kinetic energy of the molecules increases. This causes the molecules to move around more, loosening the intermolecular interactions and increasing the entropy. When enough energy is absorbed for the molecules to move freely around one another, the solid melts and becomes liquid. At the molecular level, the molecules in a liquid are still in contact and interact with each other, but they have enough kinetic energy to escape fixed positions. Liquids have more internal kinetic energy and greater entropy than solids. If enough heat is absorbed by the liquid, the kinetic energy increases until the molecules have enough speed to escape intermolecular forces and vaporize into the gas phase. Molecules in the gas phase move freely of one another and experience very little, if any, intermolecular forces. Gases are the most energetic and least ordered of the phases.

To illustrate these phase transitions, let's follow ice through the transitions from solid to liquid to gas. Ice is composed of highly organized H_2O molecules held rigidly by hydrogen bonds. The molecules have limited motion. If we increase the temperature of the ice, the molecules will eventually absorb enough heat to move around, and the organized structure of the molecules will break down as fixed hydrogen bonds are replaced with hydrogen bonds in which the molecules are *not* in fixed positions. We observe the transition as ice melting into liquid water. If we continue to increase the temperature, the kinetic energy of the molecules eventually becomes great enough for the individual molecules to overcome all hydrogen bonding and move freely. This appears to us as vaporization, or boiling of the liquid into gas. At this point the H_2O molecules zip around randomly, forming a high-entropy, chaotic swarm. All the phase transitions are summarized here.

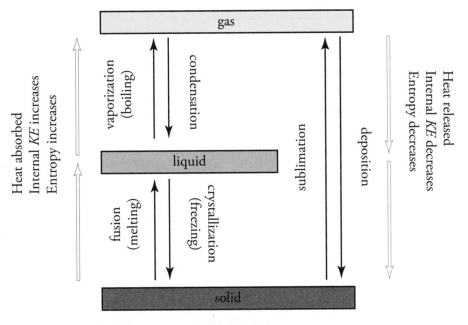

Example 7-1: Which of these phase changes releases heat energy?

A) Melting
B) Fusion
C) Condensation
D) Sublimation

Solution: Phase changes that bring molecules together (*condensation, freezing, deposition*) release heat, while phase changes that spread molecules out (*melting/fusion, vaporization, sublimation*) absorb heat. Choice C is the correct answer. (Note also that choices A and B are identical, so you know they have to be wrong no matter what.)

7.2 HEATS OF PHASE CHANGES

When matter undergoes a phase transition, energy is either absorbed or released. The amount of energy required to complete a transition is called the **heat of transition**, symbolized ΔH. For example, the amount of heat that must be absorbed to change a solid into a liquid is called the **heat of fusion**, and the energy absorbed when a liquid changes to a gas is the **heat of vaporization**. Each substance has a specific heat of transition for each phase change, and the magnitude is directly related to the strength and number of the intermolecular forces that substance experiences.

The amount of heat required to cause a change of phase depends on two things: the type of substance and the amount of substance. For example, the heat of fusion for H_2O is 6.0 kJ/mol. So, if we wanted to melt a 2 mol sample of ice (at 0°C), 12 kJ of heat would need to be supplied. The heat of vaporization for H_2O is about 41 kJ/mol, so vaporizing a 2 mol sample of liquid water (at 100°C) would require 82 kJ of heat. If that 2 mol sample of steam (at 100°C) condensed back to liquid, 82 kJ of heat would be released. In general, the amount of heat, q, accompanying a phase transition is given by

$$q = n \times \Delta H_{\text{phase change}}$$

where n is the number of moles of the substance. If ΔH and q are positive, heat is absorbed; if ΔH and q are negative, heat is released.

Example 7-2: The melting point of iron is 1530°C, and its heat of fusion is 64 cal/g. How much heat would be required to completely melt a 50 g chunk of iron at 1530°C?

Solution: Since the heat of transition is given in units of cal/g, we can simply multiply it by the given mass

$$q = m \times \Delta H_{\text{fusion}} = 50 \text{ g} \times 64 \text{ cal/g} = 3200 \text{ cal}$$

By the way, a **calorie** is, by definition, the amount of heat required to raise the temperature of 1 gram of water by 1°C. The SI unit of heat (and of all forms of energy) is the **joule**. Here's the conversion between joules and calories: 1 cal ≈ 4.2 J. (The popular term *calorie*—the one most of us are concerned with day to day when we eat—is actually a kilocalorie [10^3 cal] and is sometimes written as Calorie [with a capital C]).

Example 7-3: What happens when a container of liquid water (holding 100 moles of H_2O) at 0°C completely freezes? (Note: $\Delta H_{\text{fusion}} = 6$ kJ/mol, and $\Delta H_{\text{vap}} = 41$ kJ/mol.)

A) 600 kJ of heat is absorbed.
B) 600 kJ of heat is released.
C) 4100 kJ of heat is absorbed.
D) 4100 kJ of heat is released.

Solution: In order for ice to melt, it must absorb heat; therefore, the reverse process—water freezing into ice—must *release* heat. This eliminates choices A and C. The heat of transition from liquid to solid is $-\Delta H_{\text{fusion}}$, so in this case the heat of transition is $q = (100 \text{ mol})(-6 \text{ kJ/mol}) = -600$ kJ, so choice B is the answer.

7.3 CALORIMETRY

In between phase changes, matter can absorb or release energy without undergoing transition. We observe this as an increase or a decrease in the temperature of a substance. When a sample is undergoing a phase change, it absorbs or releases heat *without* a change in temperature, so when we talk about a temperature change, we are considering only cases where the phase doesn't change. One of the most important facts about physical changes of matter is this (and it will bear repeating):

> When a substance absorbs or releases heat, one of two things can happen: either its temperature changes *or* it will undergo a phase change *but not both at the same time.*

The amount of heat absorbed or released by a sample is proportional to its change in temperature. The constant of proportionality is called the substance's **heat capacity,** C, which is the product of its **specific heat,** c, and its mass, m; that is, $C = mc$. We can write the equation $q = C\Delta T$ in this more explicit form:

$$q = mc\Delta T$$

where

q = heat added to (or released by) a sample
m = mass of the sample
c = specific heat of the substance
ΔT = temperature change

A substance's specific heat is an *intrinsic* property of that substance and tells us how resistant it is to changing its temperature. For example, the specific heat of liquid water is 1 calorie per gram·°C. (This is actually the definition of a **calorie**: the amount of heat required to raise the temperature of 1 gram of water by 1°C.) The specific heat of copper, however, is much less: 0.09 cal/g·°C. So, if we had a 1 g sample of water and a 1 g sample of copper and each absorbed 10 calories of heat, the resulting changes in the temperatures would be

$$\Delta T_{water} = \frac{q}{mc_{water}} \qquad\qquad \Delta T_{copper} = \frac{q}{mc_{copper}}$$

$$= \frac{10 \text{ cal}}{(1 \text{ g})(1\frac{\text{cal}}{\text{g·}^\circ\text{C}})} \qquad\qquad = \frac{10 \text{ cal}}{(1 \text{ g})(0.09\frac{\text{cal}}{\text{g·}^\circ\text{C}})}$$

$$= 10^\circ\text{C} \qquad\qquad\qquad = 111^\circ\text{C}$$

That's a big difference! So, while it's true that the temperature change is proportional to the heat absorbed, it's *inversely* proportional to the substance's heat capacity. A substance like water, with a relatively high specific heat, will undergo a smaller change in temperature than a substance (like copper) with a lower specific heat.

A few notes:

1) The specific heat of a substance also depends upon phase. For example, the specific heat of ice is different from that of liquid water.
2) The SI unit for energy is the joule, not the calorie. You may see specific heats (and heat capacities) given in terms of joules rather than calories. Remember, the conversion between joules and calories is: 1 cal $\approx$ 4.2 J.
3) Specific heats may also be given in terms of kelvins rather than degrees Celsius; that is, you may see the specific heat of water, say, given as 4.2 J/g·K rather than 4.2 J/g·°C. However, since the size of a Celsius degree is the same as a kelvin (that is, if two temperatures differ by 1°C, they also differ by 1 K), the numerical value of the specific heat won't be any different if kelvins are used.

Example 7-4: The specific heat of tungsten is 0.03 cal/g·°C. If a 50-gram sample of tungsten absorbs 100 calories of heat, what will be the change in temperature of the sample?

Solution: From the equation $q = mc\Delta T$, we find that

$$\Delta T = \frac{q}{mc} = \frac{100 \text{ cal}}{(50 \text{ g})(0.03 \text{ cal/g·°C})} = \frac{2}{3/100} \text{°C} = 67 \text{°C}$$

Example 7-5: Equal amounts of heat are absorbed by 10 g solid samples of four different metals, aluminum, lead, tin, and iron. Of the four, which will exhibit the *smallest* change in temperature?

A) Aluminum (specific heat = 0.9 J/g·K)
B) Lead (specific heat = 0.13 J/g·K)
C) Tin (specific heat = 0.23 J/g·K)
D) Iron (specific heat = 0.45 J/g·K)

Solution: Since q and m are constant, ΔT is inversely proportional to c. So, the substance with the greatest specific heat will undergo the smallest change in temperature. Of the metals listed, aluminum (choice A) has the greatest specific heat.

Example 7-6: A researcher attempts to determine the specific heat of a substance by gradually heating a sample of it over time and measuring the temperature change. His first trial fails because it produces no significant change in temperature. Which changes to his experimental procedure would be most effective in producing a larger temperature change in his second trial?

A) Increasing the mass of the sample and increasing the heat input
B) Increasing the mass of the sample and decreasing the heat input
C) Decreasing the mass of the sample and increasing the heat input
D) Decreasing the mass of the sample and decreasing the heat input

Solution: Since $\Delta T = q/mc$, to increase ΔT, the researcher should increase q and decrease m. *(Intuitively, adding more heat to a smaller sample should result in a greater temperature increase.)* Therefore, the answer is C.

Example 7-7: Molecules that experience strong intermolecular forces tend to have high specific heats. Of the following molecules, which one is likely to have the highest specific heat?

A) CH_4
B) $(CH_3)_4Si$
C) CO
D) CH_3OH

Solution: We're looking for the molecule with the strongest intermolecular forces. Choices A and B are eliminated because these are nonpolar molecules that only experience weak London dispersion forces. Methanol (choice D) is a better choice than carbon monoxide (choice C), because methanol will experience hydrogen bonding while carbon monoxide experiences only weak dipole forces. Therefore, choice D is the answer.

7.4 PHASE TRANSITION DIAGRAM/HEATING CURVE

Let's consider the complete range of phase changes from solid to liquid to gas. The process in this direction requires the input of heat. As heat is added to the solid, its temperature increases until it reaches its melting point. At that point, absorbed heat is used to change the phase to liquid, not to increase the temperature. Once the sample has been completely melted, additional heat again causes its temperature to rise, until the boiling point is reached. At that point, absorbed heat is used to change the phase to gas, not to increase the temperature. Once the sample has been completely vaporized, additional heat again causes its temperature to rise. We can summarize all this with a **phase transition diagram**, also known as a **heating curve**, which plots the temperature of the sample versus the amount of heat absorbed. The figure below is a typical heating curve.

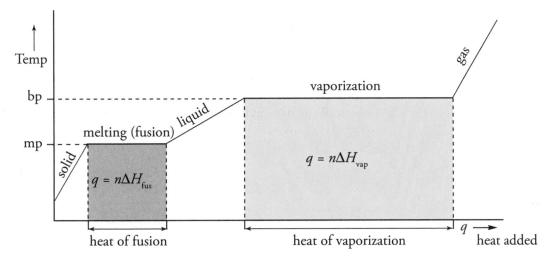

7.4

The horizontal axis represents the amount of heat added, and the vertical axis is the corresponding temperature of the substance. Notice the flat lines when the substance reaches its melting point (mp) and boiling point (bp). *During a phase transition, the temperature of the substance does not change.* Also, the greater the value for the heat of transition, the longer the flat line. A substance's heat of vaporization is always greater than its heat of fusion. The sloped lines show how the temperature changes (within a phase) as heat is added. Since $\Delta T = q/C$, the slopes of the non-flat lines are equal to $1/C$, the reciprocal of the substance's heat capacity in that phase.

Example 7-8: How much heat (in calories) is necessary to raise the temperature of 2 g of solid H_2O from 0°C to 85°C? (*Note:* Heat of fusion for water = 80 cal/g and the specific heat of water is 1 cal/g-°C.)

A) 85 cal
B) 165 cal
C) 170 cal
D) 330 cal

Solution: There are two steps here: (1) melt the ice at 0°C to liquid water at 0°C, and (2) heat the water from 0°C to 85°C.

$$\begin{aligned}
q_{total} &= q_1 + q_2 \\
&= m\Delta H_{fusion} + mc_{water}\Delta T \\
&= (2\ g)(80\ cal/g) + (2\ g)(1\ cal/g\,°C)(85\,°C) \\
&= (160\ cal) + (170\ cal) \\
&= 330\ cal
\end{aligned}$$

The correct answer is D.

Example 7-9: Given that each of the following solutions is at equilibrium with its environment, which solution should have the lowest temperature at 1 atm?

A) A solution that is 1% ice and 99% liquid water
B) A solution that is 50% ice and 50% liquid water
C) A solution that is 99% ice and 1% liquid water
D) All these solutions will have the same temperature

Solution: As long as there is any amount of ice and liquid water coexisting at equilibrium, the temperature must be 0°C at 1 atm. Therefore, D is the answer.

Phase Diagrams

The phase of a substance doesn't depend just on the temperature, it also depends on the pressure. For example, even at high temperatures, a substance can be squeezed into the liquid phase if the pressure is high enough, and at low temperature, a substance can enter the gas phase if that pressure is low enough. A substance's **phase diagram** shows how its phases are determined by temperature and pressure. The figure below is a generic example of a phase diagram.

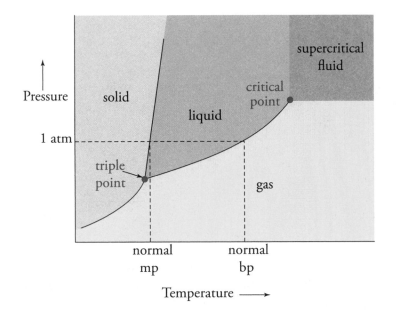

The boundary lines between phases represent points at which the two phases are in equilibrium. For example, a glass of liquid water at 0°C containing ice cubes is a two-phase system, and if its temperature and pressure were plotted in a phase diagram, it would be on the solid-liquid boundary line. Crossing a boundary line implies a phase transition. Notice that the solid phase is favored at low temperatures and high pressures, while the gas phase is favored at high temperatures and low pressures.

If we draw a horizontal line at the "1 atm" pressure level, the temperature at the point where this line crosses the solid-liquid boundary is the substance's **normal melting point**, and the temperature at the point where the line crosses the liquid-gas boundary is the **normal boiling point**.

The **triple point** is the temperature and pressure at which all three phases exist simultaneously in equilibrium, and therefore all phase changes are happening simultaneously.

The **critical point** marks the end of the liquid-gas boundary. Beyond this point, the substance displays properties of both a liquid (such as high density) and a gas (such as low viscosity). If a substance is in this state—where the liquid and gas phases are no longer distinct—it's called a **supercritical fluid**, and no amount of increased pressure can force the substance back into its liquid phase.

The Phase Diagram for Water

Water is the most common of a handful of substances that are denser in the liquid phase than in the solid phase. As a result, the solid-liquid boundary line in the phase diagram for water has a slightly *negative* slope, as opposed to the usual positive slope for most other substances. Compare these diagrams:

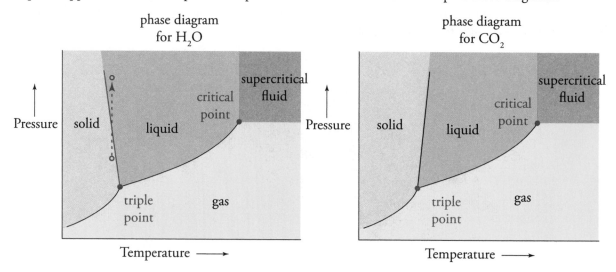

For H_2O, an increase in pressure at constant temperature can favor the *liquid* phase, not the solid phase as would be the case for most other substances (like CO_2, for example). You are probably already familiar with the following phenomenon: as the blade of an ice skate bearing all of the weight of the skater contacts the ice, the pressure increases, melting the ice under the blade and allowing the skate to glide over the liquid water. (The dashed arrow in the phase diagram for water above depicts this effect.) As the skater moves across the ice, each blade continually generates a thin layer of liquid water that refreezes as the blade passes. (This is also the reason why glaciers move.) The properties of CO_2 don't allow for skating because solid CO_2 will never turn to liquid when the pressure is increased. (And now you know why solid CO_2 is called *dry ice*!)

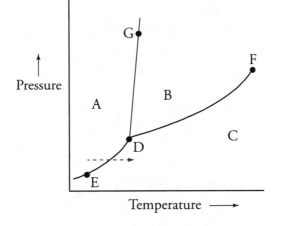

Example 7-10: In which region of the diagram above is the substance in the gas phase?

A)   A
B)   B
C)   C
D)   G

Solution: The gas phase is favored at high temperatures and low pressure, so we know that region C represents the gas phase.

Example 7-11: In which part of the diagram is gas in equilibrium with liquid?

A)   Along line ED
B)   Along line DG
C)   Along line DF
D)   In region B

Solution: The liquid phase is represented by region B and the gas phase by region C. Therefore, an equilibrium between liquid and gas phases is represented by a point on the boundary between regions B and C. This boundary is the "line" DF, choice C.

Example 7-12: The dashed arrow in the diagram indicates what type of phase transition?

A)   Evaporation
B)   Crystallization
C)   Deposition
D)   Sublimation

Solution: The arrow shows a substance in the solid phase (region A) moving directly to the gaseous phase (region C) without melting first. The phase transition from solid to gas is called sublimation, choice D.

Chapter 7 Summary

- Changes in pressure and/or temperature of a substance can induce changes in phase.

- The three important phases are (in order of low-to-high entropy and low-to-high internal energy) solid, liquid, and gas.

- Specific heat (c) is an intrinsic property that defines how resistant a substance is to temperature change.

- The change in temperature associated with the input or extraction of heat when phase is uncharged is given by $q = mc\Delta T$, where c is the specific heat of a substance and m is the amount (either mass or moles, depending on c).

- Heat capacity (C) is given by $C = mc$, where m is the mass of the sample. Heat capacity is a proportionality constant that defines how much heat is required to change the temperature of a sample by 1°C.

- A substance cannot simultaneously undergo a phase change and a temperature change.

- The heat associated with a phase change is given by $q = n\Delta H_{phase\ change}$, where n is the number of moles of substance (or mass if ΔH is given in energy/mass).

- Lines on a phase diagram correspond to equilibria between phases and phase transitions. The intersection of all three lines on a phase diagram is known as the triple point, and represents equilibrium between all three phases.

- The phase diagram of water is unique in that its solid/liquid equilibrium line has a negative slope. This accounts for the fact that ice melts under increased pressure, and why the density of ice is less than that of liquid water.

CHAPTER 7 FREESTANDING PRACTICE QUESTIONS

1. Which of the following correctly describe(s) the physical properties of water?

    I.   The hydrogen bonds in water result in a lower boiling point than H_2S.
    II. Water has a high specific heat due to the hydrogen bonding between molecules.
    III. As pressure increases liquid water is favored over solid water.

    A) II only
    B) III only
    C) II and III only
    D) I, II and III

2. As a substance goes from the gas phase to the solid phase, heat is:

    A) absorbed, internal energy decreases, and entropy decreases.
    B) released, internal energy increases, and entropy decreases.
    C) released, internal energy decreases, and entropy decreases.
    D) released, internal energy decreases, and entropy increases.

3. In the following phase transition diagram, Substance X is in the solid phase during Segment A and in the gas phase during Segment C. What process is occurring during Segment B?

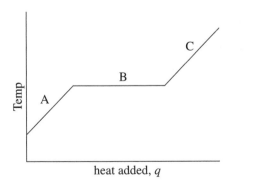

heat added, q

    A) The substance is warming.
    B) The substance is cooling.
    C) Sublimation
    D) Condensation

4. Denver is at a higher altitude than Los Angeles and therefore the atmospheric pressure is lower in Denver than in Los Angeles. Compared to Los Angeles, the melting point of water in Denver will be:

    A) higher.
    B) lower.
    C) the same.
    D) undetermined from the information given.

5. At 1 atm, deionized water can remain a liquid at temperatures down to –42°C. If a foreign body is added to the supercooled liquid, it will immediately turn into ice. Which of the following is true about this process?

    A) The reaction is exothermic.
    B) Tap water could also be supercooled to –42°C.
    C) The transformation of a supercooled fluid to a solid is nonspontaneous.
    D) Water's unique phase diagram allows it to be supercooled.

6. A pot containing 0.5 L of water at sea level is brought to 100°C. It is insulated around its sides to minimize heat loss to the environment, and heat is applied at the bottom of the container at a rate of 6 kJ/min over 3 minutes. What is the resulting temperature of the water? (ΔH_{vap} = 40.7 kJ/mol; $c(g)$ = 1.9 kJ/kg · °C; $c(l)$ = 4.2 kJ/kg · °C)

    A) 115°C
    B) 108°C
    C) 104°C
    D) 100°C

CHAPTER 7 PRACTICE PASSAGE

Lyophilization, or freeze drying, is a technique used to remove water from samples. Lyophilization uses sublimation to convert frozen, solid water directly to water vapor. This technique offers advantages over liquid-solvent removal techniques in that it can be performed at low temperatures, resulting in minimal damage to heat-sensitive samples.

A chamber containing the sample solution is attached to the lyophilizer, which freezes the sample at a temperature less than 0°C and then applies a vacuum, generally holding a pressure less than 0.006 atm. Under these conditions the frozen water sublimes and water vapor is pulled from the sample chamber into a condenser held at 50°C, where it is refrozen and held immobile.

The phase diagram for water is shown below, with its unique negatively sloped equilibrium line between the solid and liquid phase. At low pressures the solid phase of water is favored as long as any solute in the water is reasonably dilute. However, the freezing point of water decreases as the concentration of solute is increased. If concentrated enough, the sample can melt instead of sublime when pressure is decreased. In addition, volatile solvents often cannot be removed from the chamber by the condenser as their freezing point at low pressures is below −50°C. Volatile solvents remaining in the gaseous environment can compound the impurity of the remaining water, favoring the liquid phase even more.

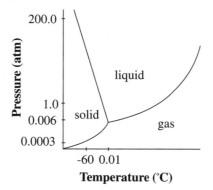

Figure 1 Phase diagram of water

1. The addition of which of the following substances is most likely to result in the melting of a sample during lyophilization?

A) $(CH_3)_2CHOH$
B) CH_3CH_2COOH
C) $CH_3CH_2OCH_2CH_3$
D) $CH_3(CH_2)_4OH$

2. If the temperature inside the chamber is −60°C, what pressure must the chamber be at in order for the sublimation reaction to be at equilibrium?

A) 3×10^{-4} atm
B) 3×10^{-3} atm
C) 1 atm
D) 125 atm

3. Lyophilization would most likely be employed industrially in which of the following separations?

A) Salicylic acid dissolved in methanol
B) An enzyme in aqueous solution
C) NaCl in water
D) A small molecular drug dissolved in dichloromethane

4. Sublimation of water inside the sample chamber causes the temperature of the chamber to:

A) increase.
B) decrease.
C) stay the same.
D) change in a manner dependent on the identity of the solvent.

5. The heat of sublimation of water is 46 kJ/mol. If heat is transferred to the sample by the environment at a rate of 0.1 kJ/min, approximately how long will it take to lyophilize 40 cm³ of frozen water (density = 0.91 g/mL) ?

A) 7.7 hours
B) 15.3 hours
C) 77.0 hours
D) 153.0 hours

SOLUTIONS TO CHAPTER 7 FREESTANDING PRACTICE QUESTIONS

1. **C** Since water experiences hydrogen bonding, more energy is required to boil water compared with SH_2, which leads to a higher boiling point, making Item I false and eliminating choice D. Since temperature is a measure of molecular motion, and hydrogen bonds bind molecules together, making this motion more difficult, hydrogen-bonded materials will require more energy to increase T and thus have high specific heats. Item II is true and choice B can be eliminated. The negative slope of the line between the solid and liquid phase on the phase diagram of water indicates that at higher pressures, liquid water is favored over solid, making Item III correct and C the best answer choice.

2. **C** As a substance undergoes deposition, it becomes a much more ordered substance, decreasing entropy (eliminate choice D). In addition, heat will be released (eliminate choice A) because the potential energy of the substance decreases (eliminate choice B).

3. **C** Substance X is changing from a solid to a gas during Segment B. This is an example of sublimation. Note that choices A and B cannot be correct answer choices because the temperature of Substance X remains constant during Segment B. Condensation occurs when a gas becomes a liquid, so choice D is eliminated.

4. **A** On a P vs. T phase diagram of water, the solid-liquid equilibrium line has a negative slope for water. Water's melting point increases with decreasing external pressure. Therefore, in Denver the melting point of water is higher than in Los Angeles.

5. **A** Upon nucleation with a foreign body, supercooled water will transition from liquid to solid phase. This phase transition (crystallization) requires heat to be released since intermolecular interactions are formed. Choice B is eliminated because tap water contains many dissolved particles that can serve as sites of nucleation. Choice C is incorrect because the supercooled fluids are only kinetically stabilized against freezing, and their transformation to a solid form is thermodynamically spontaneous. Since pressure remains constant, the negative sloped solid-liquid equilibrium line in water's phase diagram does not play a role in supercooling, eliminating Choice D.

6. **D** The addition of 6 kJ/min for three minutes imparts 18 kJ of heat to the sample. However, since the ΔH_{vap} of water is 40.7 kJ/mol, and 0.5 L is roughly 28 mol (1 L of $H_2O \approx 55$ mol), there is nowhere near enough heat provided to vaporize the entire sample. As such all the heat given to the sample is going toward vaporization and not toward increasing temperature. The temperature will remain constant at 100°C.

SOLUTIONS TO CHAPTER 7 PRACTICE PASSAGE

1. **C**   The passage states that volatile chemicals cannot be used in samples subjected to lyophilization because they will hinder sublimation and favor the liquid phase through melting. This is because these compounds have a high vapor pressure and cannot be removed from the system by the condenser. Choices A, B, and D are all hydrogen donors and acceptors. Choice C, diethyl ether, can only act as a hydrogen bond acceptor. Therefore, it has the weakest intermolecular forces and is the most volatile.

2. **A**   On a P vs. T diagram, sublimation equilibrium is indicated by the line separating the solid and vapor phases. On the graph in Figure 1, it is shown that at $-60°C$, the solid/gas line is at $P = 0.0003$ or 3×10^{-4} atm.

3. **B**   Both dichloromethane and methanol are removed as liquids at reasonably low temperatures and have freezing points far lower than water. This eliminates choices A and D. The passage states that one of the major advantages to lyophilization is that it can be performed at low temperatures, and therefore preserve the activity of heat-sensitive samples. NaCl is a salt that is stable at high temperatures, whereas enzymes are proteins that denature at high temperatures. Therefore, lyophilization is best suited as a means to remove water from aqueous protein solutions.

4. **B**   Sublimation is an endothermic reaction, requiring heat input. As this reaction removes heat from the surroundings, it lowers the temperature of the surroundings, in this case, the reaction chamber. This is very similar to sweat cooling the body as it evaporates off of the skin (also an endothermic process).

5. **B**   40 cm^3 of ice is 36 g or 2 moles of water. The heat required to sublimate this sample is 46 kJ/mol(2 mol) = 92 kJ. If heat is transferred at 0.1 kJ/min, then 920 minutes are required. Dividing 920 min by 60 min/hour gives just over 15 hours. Overall:

$$Time = (40\,cm^3)\left(\frac{0.91g}{mL}\right)\left(\frac{molH_2O}{18g}\right)\left(\frac{46\,kJ}{mol}\right)\left(\frac{min}{0.1\,kJ}\right)\left(\frac{hour}{60\,min}\right)$$

$$Time \approx (40\,cm^3)\left(\frac{0.9g}{mL}\right)\left(\frac{molH_2O}{18g}\right)\left(\frac{45\,kJ}{mol}\right)\left(\frac{min}{0.1\,kJ}\right)\left(\frac{hour}{60\,min}\right)$$

$$Time \approx 15 \text{ hours}$$

Chapter 8
Gases

8.1 GASES AND THE KINETIC-MOLECULAR THEORY

Unlike the condensed phases of matter (solids and liquids), **gases** have no fixed volume. A gas will fill all the available space in a container. Gases are *far* more compressible than solids or liquids, and their densities are very low (roughly 1 kg/m³ at standard temperature and pressure), about three to four orders of magnitude less than solids and liquids. But the most striking difference between a gas and a solid or liquid is that the molecules of a gas are free to move over large distances.

The most important properties of a gas are its **pressure**, **volume**, and **temperature**. How these macroscopic properties are related to each other can be derived from some basic assumptions concerning the *microscopic* behavior of gas molecules. These assumptions are the foundation of the **kinetic-molecular theory**.

Kinetic-molecular theory, a model for describing the behavior of gases, is based on the following assumptions:

1) The molecules of a gas are so small compared to the average spacing between them that the molecules themselves take up essentially no volume.

2) The molecules of a gas are in constant motion, moving in straight lines at constant speeds and in random directions between collisions. The collisions of the molecules with the walls of the container define the **pressure** of the gas (the average force exerted per unit area), and all collisions—molecules striking the walls and each other—are *elastic* (that is, the total kinetic energy is the same after the collision as it was before).

3) Since each molecule moves at a constant speed between collisions and the collisions are elastic, the molecules of a gas experience no intermolecular forces.

4) The molecules of a gas span a distribution of speeds, and the average kinetic energy of the molecules is directly proportional to the absolute temperature (the temperature in kelvins) of the sample: $KE_{avg} \propto T$.

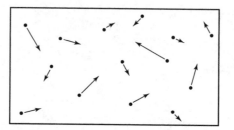

A gas that satisfies all these requirements is said to be an **ideal gas.** Most real gases behave like ideal gases under ordinary conditions, so the results that follow from the kinetic-molecular theory can be applied to real gases.

Units of Volume, Temperature, and Pressure

Volume

The SI unit for volume is the cubic meter (m³), but in chemistry, the **cubic centimeter** (cm³ or **cc**) and **liter** (**L**) are commonly used. One cubic meter is equal to one thousand liters.

$$1 \text{ cm}^3 = 1 \text{ cc} = 1 \text{ mL} \quad \text{and} \quad 1 \text{ m}^3 = 1000 \text{ L}$$

Temperature

Temperature may be expressed in degrees Fahrenheit, degrees Celsius, or in kelvins (not degrees Kelvin). In scientific work, the Celsius scale is popular, where water freezes at 0°C and boils at 100°C (at standard atmospheric pressure). However, the "proper" unit for expressing temperatures is the kelvin (K), and this is the one we use when talking about gases (because of assumption #4 stated above for the kinetic-molecular theory). The relationship between kelvins and degrees Celsius is simple:

$$T \text{ (in K)} = T \text{ (in °C)} + 273.15$$

When dealing with gases, the best unit for expressing temperature is the kelvin (K). This is an absolute temperature scale whereby zero kelvin (0 K) defines a point of zero entropy (see Chapter 6) where molecular motion is at a minimum. From a practical perspective, this avoids the issue of calculations involving negative temperatures, so all of the gas laws equations on the MCAT require the use of absolute temperatures.

Pressure

Since pressure is defined as force per unit area, the SI unit for pressure is the **pascal** (abbreviated **Pa**), where $1 \text{ Pa} = 1 \text{ N/m}^2$. The unit is inconveniently small for normal calculations involving gases (for example, a nickel sitting on a table exerts about 140 Pa of pressure), so several alternative units for pressure are usually used.

At sea level, atmospheric pressure is about 101,300 pascals (or 100 kPa for MCAT math); this is 1 **atmosphere (1 atm)**. Related to the atmosphere is the **torr**, where 1 atm = 760 torr. (Therefore, 1 torr is about the same as the pressure exerted by a nickel sitting on a table.) At 0°C, 1 torr is equal to 1 **mm Hg (millimeter of mercury)**, so we generally just take 1 atm to equal 760 mm Hg:

$$1 \text{ atm} = 760 \text{ torr} = 760 \text{ mm Hg} = 101.3 \text{ kPa}$$

Standard Temperature and Pressure

Standard Temperature and Pressure (STP) means a temperature of 0°C (273.15 K) and a pressure of 1 atm.

Example 8-1: A temperature of 273°C is equivalent to:

A) −100 K
B) 0 K
C) 100 K
D) 546 K

Solution: Choice A is eliminated, because negative values are not permitted when using the Kelvin temperature scale. Since $T \text{ (in K)} = T \text{ (in °C)} + 273$, we have

$$T \text{ (in K)} = 273 + 273 = 546 \text{ K}$$

Therefore, choice D is the answer.

Example 8-2: What would be the reading of a barometer (a device used to measure pressure) filled with a liquid of lower density than Hg if at that moment another nearby Hg barometer reads 752 mm Hg?

A) Less than 752 mm
B) 752 mm
C) Greater than 752 mm
D) It depends on the compressibility of the liquid.

Solution: In a mercury barometer, the atmospheric pressure pushes a column of Hg up a tube until the weight of the column of Hg balances the upward pressure of the atmosphere; one then reads the height of the suspended Hg column in millimeters. If a less dense liquid were used, then more liquid would have to get pushed up the column before it weighed enough to balance the atmospheric pressure. The liquid column would then have a greater strength, so choice C is the correct answer.

8.2 THE IDEAL GAS LAW

The volume, temperature, and pressure of an ideal gas are related by a simple equation called the **ideal gas law.** Most real gases under ordinary conditions act very much like ideal gases, so the ideal gas law applies to most gas behavior:

> **Ideal Gas Law**
> $$PV = nRT$$

where

P = the pressure of the gas in atmospheres
V = the volume of the container in liters
n = the number of moles of the gas
R = the universal gas constant, 0.0821 L-atm/K-mol
T = the absolute temperature of the gas (that is, T in kelvins)

Questions on gas behavior typically take one of two forms. The first type of question simply gives you some facts, and you use $PV = nRT$ to determine a missing variable. In the second type, "before" and "after" scenarios are presented for which you determine the effect of changing the volume, temperature, or pressure. In this case, you apply the ideal gas law twice, once for each scenario. We'll solve a typical example of each type of question.

1. If two moles of helium at 27°C fill a 3 L balloon, what is the pressure?

Take the ideal gas law, solve it for P, then plug in the numbers (and don't forget to convert the temperature in °C to kelvin!):

$$PV = nRT$$

$$P = \frac{nRT}{V}$$

$$P = \frac{(2 \text{ mol})(0.082 \text{ L-atm/K-mol})(300 \text{ K})}{3 \text{ L}}$$

$$P = 16 \text{ atm}$$

2. Argon, at a pressure of 2 atm, fills a 100 mL vial at a temperature of 0°C. What would the pressure of the argon be if we increase the volume to 500 mL, and the temperature is 100°C?

We're not told how much argon (the number of moles, n) is in the vial, but it doesn't matter since it doesn't change. Since R is also a constant, the ratio of PV/T, which is equal to nR, remains constant. Therefore,

$$\frac{P_1 V_1}{T_1} = \frac{P_2 V_2}{T_2} \quad \Rightarrow \quad P_2 = P_1 \frac{V_1}{V_2} \frac{T_2}{T_1}$$

$$P_2 = (2 \text{ atm}) \left(\frac{0.1 \text{ L}}{0.5 \text{ L}} \right) \left(\frac{373 \text{ K}}{273 \text{ K}} \right)$$

$$P_2 = 0.55 \text{ atm}$$

P-V-T Gas Laws in Systems Where n Is Constant

As we saw in answering Question 2 above, the amount of gas often remains the same, and the n drops out (we make this assumption in the equations that follow). Our work can be simplified even further if the pressure, temperature, or volume is also held constant. (And remember: when working with the gas laws, *temperature* always means *absolute temperature* [that is, T in kelvins].)

- If the pressure is constant, $V/T = k$ (where k is a constant). Therefore, the volume is proportional to the temperature: $V \propto T$

This is known as **Charles's law.** If the pressure is to remain constant, then a gas will expand when heated and contract when cooled. If the temperature of the gas is increased, the molecules will move faster, hitting the walls of the container with more force; in order to keep the pressure the same, the frequency of the collisions would need to be reduced. This is accomplished by expanding the volume. With more available space, the molecules strike the walls less often in order to compensate for hitting them harder.

- If the temperature is constant, $PV = k$ (where k is a constant). Therefore, the pressure is inversely proportional to the volume: $P \propto 1/V$

This is known as **Boyle's law**. If the volume decreases, the molecules have less space to move around in. As a result, they'll collide with the walls of the container more often, and the pressure increases. On the other hand, if the volume of the container increases, the gas molecules have more available space and collide with the wall less often, resulting in a lower pressure.

- If the volume is constant, $P/T = k$ (where k is a constant). Therefore, the pressure is proportional to the temperature: $P \propto T$

If the temperature goes up, so does the pressure. This should make sense when you consider the origin of pressure. As the temperature increases, the molecules move faster. As a result, they strike the walls of the container surface more often and with greater speed.

Since each of the two-variable relationships reviewed above are equal to a constant as described, this means that the product or quotient will not change if we meet the specified assumptions (hold the other variables constant). This allows us to generate equations where we compare properties of a gas under two different conditions:

In a system with constant n:

At constant P: $\dfrac{V_1}{T_1} = \dfrac{V_2}{T_2}$

At constant T: $P_1V_1 = P_2V_2$

At constant V: $\dfrac{P_1}{T_1} = \dfrac{P_2}{T_2}$

If only n (which tells us the amount of gas) stays constant, we can combine Boyle's Law and Charles's Law to get the **combined gas law** (which we used to answer Question 2 above):

Combined Gas Law (constant n)
$$\frac{P_1V_1}{T_1} = \frac{P_2V_2}{T_2}$$

Example 8-3: Helium, at a pressure of 3 atm, occupies a 16 L container at a temperature of 30°C. What would be the volume of the gas if the pressure were increased to 5 atm and the temperature lowered to –20°C?

Solution: We use the combined gas law after remembering to convert the given temperatures to kelvin:

$$\frac{P_1V_1}{T_1} = \frac{P_2V_2}{T_2} \implies V_2 = V_1\frac{P_1}{P_2}\frac{T_2}{T_1} = (16\text{ L})\left(\frac{3\text{ atm}}{5\text{ atm}}\right)\left(\frac{253\text{ K}}{303\text{ K}}\right) \approx (16\text{ L})\left(\frac{3}{5}\right)\left(\frac{250\text{ K}}{300\text{ K}}\right) = 8\text{ L}$$

All of these laws follow from the ideal gas law and can be derived easily from it. They tell us what happens when n and P are constant, when n and T are constant, when n and V are constant, and in the case of the combined gas law, when n alone is constant. But what about n when P, V, and T are constant? That law of gases was proposed by Avogadro:

- If two equal-volume containers hold gas at the same pressure and temperature, then they contain the same number of particles (regardless of the identity of the gas).

Avogadro's law can be restated more broadly as **$V/n = k$** (where k is a constant). We can also determine the **standard molar volume** of an ideal gas at STP, which is the volume that one mole of a gas—any *ideal* gas*—would occupy at 0°C and 1 atm of pressure:

$$V = \frac{nRT}{P} = \frac{(1 \text{ mol})(0.0821 \text{L·atm/K·mol})(273 \text{ K})}{1 \text{ atm}} = 22.4 \text{ L}$$

To give you an idea of how much this is, 22.4 L is equal to the total volume of three basketballs.

Avogrado's law and the **standard molar volume** of a gas can be used to simplify some gas law problems. Consider the following questions:

> 3. Given the Haber process, $3 H_2(g) + N_2(g) \rightarrow 2 NH_3(g)$, if you start with 5 L of $H_2(g)$ and 4 L of $N_2(g)$ at STP, what will the volume of the three gases be when the reaction is complete?

We can answer this question by using the ideal gas law, or we can recognize that the only thing changing is n (the number of moles of each gas) and use the standard molar volume. If we further recognize that the standard molar volume is the same for all three gases, and it is this value that we'd use to convert each given volume into moles (and then vice versa), we can use the balanced equation to quickly determine the answer.

Since we need 3 L of H_2 for every 1 L of N_2, and we have 4 L of N_2 but only 5 L of H_2, H_2 will be the limiting reagent, and its volume will be zero at the end of the reaction. Since 1 L of N_2 is needed for every 3 L of H_2, we get

$$5 \text{ L of H}_2 \times \frac{1 \text{ L of N}_2}{3 \text{ L of H}_2} = 1.7 \text{ L of N}_2$$

So the amount of N_2 remaining will be $4 - 1.7 = 2.3$ L. The volume of NH_3 produced is

$$5 \text{ L of H}_2 \times \frac{2 \text{ L of NH}_3}{3 \text{ L of H}_2} = 3.3 \text{ L of NH}_3$$

Example 8-4: Three moles of oxygen gas are present in a 10 L chamber at a temperature of 25°C. Which one of the following expressions is equal to the pressure of the gas (in atm)?

A) (3)(0.08)(10)/25
B) (3)(0.08)(25)/10
C) (3)(0.08)(10)/298
D) (3)(0.08)(298)/10

Solution: Since 25°C = 298 K, the ideal gas law gives

$$P = \frac{nRT}{V} = \frac{(3)(0.08)(298)}{10} \text{ atm}$$

The answer is D.

Example 8-5: An ideal gas at 2 atm occupies a 5-liter tank. It is then transferred to a new tank of volume 12 liters. If temperature is held constant throughout, what is the new pressure?

Solution: Since n and T are constants, we can use Boyle's law to find

$$P_1 V_1 = P_2 V_2 \quad \Rightarrow \quad P_2 = P_1 \frac{V_1}{V_2} = (2 \text{ atm}) \frac{5 \text{ L}}{12 \text{ L}} = \frac{5}{6} \text{ atm}$$

Example 8-6: A 6-liter container holds $H_2(g)$ at a temperature of 400 K and a pressure of 3 atm. If the temperature is increased to 600 K, what will be the pressure?

Solution: Since n and V are constants, we can write

$$\frac{P_1}{T_1} = \frac{P_2}{T_2} \quad \Rightarrow \quad P_2 = P_1 \frac{T_2}{T_1} = (3 \text{ atm}) \frac{600 \text{ K}}{400 \text{ K}} = 4.5 \text{ atm}$$

Example 8-7: How many atoms of helium are present in 11.2 liters of the gas at $P = 1$ atm and $T = 273$ K?

A) 3.01×10^{23}
B) 6.02×10^{23}
C) 1.20×10^{24}
D) Cannot be determined from the information given

Solution: $P = 1$ atm and $T = 273$ K define STP, so 1 mole of an ideal gas would occupy 22.4 L. A volume of 11.2 L is exactly half this so it must correspond to a 0.5 mole sample. Since 1 mole of helium contains 6.02×10^{23} atoms, 0.5 mole contains half this many: 3.01×10^{23} (choice A).

8.3 DEVIATIONS FROM IDEAL-GAS BEHAVIOR

Let's review two of the assumptions that were listed for the kinetic-molecular theory:

1) The particles of an ideal gas experience no intermolecular forces.
2) The volume of the individual particles of an ideal gas is negligible compared to the volume of the gas container.

Under some conditions, namely high pressures and low temperatures, these assumptions don't hold up very well, and the laws for ideal gases don't rigorously apply to real gases.

To determine the effect of non-ideality on gases on a macroscopic level, work though the following thought experiments, which examine each assumption above independently:

1) *No intermolecular forces:*

   Imagine blowing up a balloon to a given volume with an ideal gas. Now, fix the volume of the container and allow the gas to behave as a real gas with strongly attractive intermolecular forces (e.g., like water vapor would have). How will the pressure change? Remember that the number of collisions gas particles have with the container walls (and their momentum) determines pressure. While the particles in a real gas have attractive intermolecular forces, they do not have the same attractive forces with the walls. Increased particle interactions therefore lead to fewer collisions with the walls of the container, and the collisions that do occur will involve a smaller transfer of momentum than they would have if the gas were ideal and all collisions perfectly elastic. The resulting pressure of the real gas is therefore smaller than if the gas were ideal, or $P_{real} < P_{ideal}$.

2) *Volumeless particles:*

   Imagine blowing up a balloon with an ideal gas somewhere half-way through the atmosphere of Jupiter (with its high pressures), then fix the pressure of the ideal gas system after it equilibrates with external pressure. Now, instead of the ideal volumeless particles, give the individual gas particles finite volumes. How does the volume of the gas change? The tricky part here is that the volume of a gas is defined as the free space the particles have in which to move around. For an ideal gas this volume is simply the volume of the container, since there is no volume taken up by individual particles. However, at high pressures the volume occupied by each gas particle becomes a greater proportion of the gas sample, so it is no longer negligible, and reduces the free space available for particle movement. The overall effect is to decrease the volume, making $V_{real} < V_{ideal}$.

From these two thought experiments we see that the attractive forces between particles cause a decrease in pressure if the volume of the container is fixed, and accounting for particle volume causes a decrease in free space (system volume) if the pressure is fixed. As these two variables interact with many others in a real system, we can sometimes see deviations from the general principles outlined here, especially at exceedingly high pressures.[1] However, complex situations like this are beyond the scope of the MCAT, so we will focus our analysis on the deviations as described above.

---

[1]   For example, at pressures > 300 atm, gas particles are pushed so close together that they begin to repel one another, which can result in an increase in the volume of real gases over what would be predicted by the ideal gas law.

8.3

To make accurate predictions about the deviations real gases show from ideal-gas behavior, the ideal gas law must be altered. The **van der Waals equation** includes terms to account for the differences in the observed behavior of real gases and calculated properties of ideal gases, while maintaining the same form as the ideal gas law:

---

van der Waals Equation

$$\left(P + \frac{an^2}{V^2} \right)(V - nb) = nRT$$

The an^2/V^2 term serves as a correction for the intermolecular forces that generally result in lower pressures for real gases, while the nb term corrects for the physical volume that the individual particles occupy in a real gas. Both a and b are known as van der Waals constants and are generally larger for gases that experience greater intermolecular forces (a) and have larger molecular weights, and therefore volumes (b).

To illustrate the impact of intermolecular forces on real gas pressure, let's compare the pressures of two moles of oxygen and two moles of water, each in separate 5 L containers at a moderate temperature (500 K). Using the ideal gas law, we predict the following:

$$P_{\text{ideal}} = \frac{nRT}{V} = \frac{2 \text{ moles} \times 0.0821 \text{ L·atm/mol·K} \times 500 \text{ K}}{5 \text{L}} = 16.4 \text{ atm}$$

To use the van der Waals equation to predict the actual pressures, we can rearrange and solve for P.

$$P = \left(\frac{nRT}{V - nb} \right) - \left(\frac{an^2}{V^2} \right)$$

Therefore for oxygen (where a = 1.34 atm·L^2/mol^2 and b = 0.0318 L/mol):

$$P_{O_2} = \left(\frac{2 \text{ mol} \times 0.0821 \text{ L·atm/mol·K} \times 500 \text{ K}}{5 \text{ L} - 2 \text{ mol} \times 0.0318 \text{ L/mol}} \right) - \left(\frac{1.34 \text{ atm·L}^2/\text{mol}^2 \times (2 \text{ mol})^2}{(5 \text{ L})^2} \right)$$

$$= 16.6 \text{ atm} - 0.2 \text{ atm} = 16.4 \text{ atm}$$

Notice that the pressure, due to oxygen's lack of substantial intermolecular forces, is effectively the same as was predicted by the ideal gas law. If we select a gas with significantly stronger intermolecular forces, the deviation from ideal gas behavior becomes more pronounced. For instance, the van der Waals "a" constant for water is significantly higher than that of oxygen due to water's ability to hydrogen bond (a = 5.47 atm·L^2/mol^2 and b = 0.0305 L/mol).

$$P_{H_2O} = \left(\frac{2 \text{ mol} \times 0.0821 \text{ L·atm/mol·K} \times 500 \text{ K}}{5 \text{ L} - 2 \text{ mol} \times 0.0305 \text{ L/mol}} \right) - \left(\frac{5.47 \text{ atm·L}^2/\text{mol}^2 \times (2 \text{ mol})^2}{(5 \text{ L})^2} \right)$$

$$= 16.6 \text{ atm} - 0.9 \text{ atm} = 15.7 \text{ atm}$$

This represents a 4% decrease in pressure from that predicted by the ideal gas law.

To underscore the concept that gases behave more ideally at higher temperatures, if we increase the temperature of the system for any gas, the first term in the van der Waals equation approaches the pressure of the ideal gas while the second term remains unchanged. For example, if the temperature of our systems above is increased by 100 K (to 600 K), two moles of an ideal gas would exert 19.7 atm of pressure, while the van der Waals equation predicts pressures of 19.7 atm and 19.1 atm for oxygen and water, respectively. Therefore, we can see that at increased temperature the real gas (H_2O) behaves more ideally since it now deviates by only 3% from the pressure predicted by the ideal gas law.

So conceptually, why do higher pressures and lower temperatures cause larger deviations from ideal behavior? As pressure increases, gas particles become closer to one another. This accentuates the effects of attractive intermolecular forces, causing a decrease in observed pressure ($P_{real} < P_{ideal}$). Similarly, at low temperatures intermolecular forces become more important, and when taken to an extreme, cause condensation to occur. Liquids aren't very ideal gases. In addition, when gas particles are packed closer to one another at high pressures, particle volume of the gas itself begins to limit the free space in which the gas particles can move ($V_{real} < V_{ideal}$). However under extremely high pressure, these particles can begin to repel one another leading to an increase in volume.

To summarize and focus on MCAT-relevance, those gases that behave most ideally have the weakest intermolecular forces and the smallest molecular weights (and volumes). Furthermore, by maintaining conditions of high temperature and low pressure, the potential interactions between particles are minimized and particle volume remains insignificant compared to the container size, helping to favor more ideal behavior for all gases.

Example 8-8: Of the following, which gas would likely *deviate* the most from ideal behavior at high pressure and low temperature?

A) $He(g)$
B) $H_2(g)$
C) $O_2(g)$
D) $H_2O(g)$

Solution: Since H_2O molecules will experience hydrogen bonding, they feel significantly stronger intermolecular forces than the other gases do. Therefore, of the choices given, $H_2O(g)$ will deviate the most from ideal behavior at high pressure and low temperature.

Example 8-9: Of the following, which gas would behave most like an ideal gas if all were at the same temperature and pressure?

A) $O_2(g)$
B) $CH_4(g)$
C) $Ar(g)$
D) $Cl_2(g)$

Solution: The molecules of a perfect (ideal) gas take up zero volume, so the gas in this list that will behave most like an ideal gas will be the one that takes up the smallest volume. O_2, CH_4, and Cl_2 are all polyatomic molecules that occupy more space than atomic argon. Therefore, choice C is the answer.

Example 8-10: Of the following, which gas would behave most like an ideal gas if all were at the same temperature and pressure?

A) $H_2O(g)$
B) $CH_4(g)$
C) $HF(g)$
D) $NH_3(g)$

Solution: The molecules of a perfect (ideal) gas experience no intermolecular forces, so the gas in this list that will behave most like an ideal gas will be the one that has the weakest intermolecular forces. H_2O, HF, and NH_3 experience hydrogen-bonding, while CH_4 experiences only weak dispersion forces. Therefore, choice B is the answer.

Example 8-11: Under which of the following conditions does the ideal gas law give the most accurate results for a real gas?

A) Low T and low P
B) Low T and high P
C) High T and low P
D) High T and high P

Solution: Real gases can never behave as true ideal gases because 1) their molecules occupy space, and 2) their molecules experience attractive intermolecular forces. However, when gas molecules are spread out, these violations are minimized. The physical conditions that allow for gases to spread out are high temperature and low pressure, choice C.

8.4   DALTON'S LAW OF PARTIAL PRESSURES

Consider a mixture of, say, three gases in a single container.

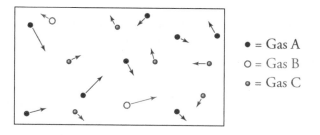

The total pressure is due to the collisions of all three types of molecules with the container walls. The pressure that the molecules of Gas A alone exert is called the **partial pressure** of Gas A, denoted by p_A. Similarly, the pressure exerted by the molecules of Gas B alone and the pressure exerted by the molecules of Gas C alone are p_B and p_C.

Dalton's law of partial pressures says that the total pressure is simply the sum of the partial pressures of all the constituent gases. In this case, then, we'd have

Dalton's Law

$$P_{tot} = p_A + p_B + p_C$$

So, if we know the partial pressures, we can determine the total pressure. We can also work backward. Knowing the total pressure, we can figure out the individual partial pressures. All that is required is the mole fraction. For example, in the diagram above, there are a total of 16 molecules: 8 of Gas A, 2 of Gas B, and 6 of Gas C. Therefore, the mole fraction of Gas A is $X_A = 8/16 = 1/2$, the mole fraction of Gas B is $X_B = 2/16 = 1/8$, and the mole fraction of Gas C is $X_C = 6/16 = 3/8$. *The partial pressure of a gas is equal to its mole fraction times the total pressure.* For example, if the total pressure in the container above is 8 atm, then

$$p_A = X_A P_{tot} = \frac{1}{2} P_{tot} = \frac{1}{2}(8 \text{ atm}) = 4 \text{ atm}$$

$$p_B = X_B P_{tot} = \frac{1}{8} P_{tot} = \frac{1}{8}(8 \text{ atm}) = 1 \text{ atm}$$

$$p_C = X_C P_{tot} = \frac{3}{8} P_{tot} = \frac{3}{8}(8 \text{ atm}) = 3 \text{ atm}$$

Example 8-12: A mixture of neon and nitrogen contains 0.5 mol Ne(g) and 2 mol $N_2(g)$. If the total pressure is 20 atm, what is the partial pressure of the neon?

Solution: The mole fraction of Ne is

$$X_{Ne} = \frac{n_{Ne}}{n_{Ne} + n_{N_2}} = \frac{0.5}{(0.5 + 2)} = \frac{0.5}{2.5} = \frac{1}{5}$$

Therefore,

$$p_{Ne} = X_{Ne} P_{tot} = \frac{1}{5} P_{tot} = \frac{1}{5}(20 \text{ atm}) = 4 \text{ atm}$$

Example 8-13: A vessel contains a mixture of three gases: A, B, and C. There is twice as much A as B and half as much C as A. If the total pressure is 300 torr, what is the partial pressure of Gas C?

A) 60 torr
B) 75 torr
C) 100 torr
D) 120 torr

Solution: The question states that there is twice as much A as B, and it also says (backward) there is twice as much A as C. So the amounts of B and C are the same, and each is half the amount of A. Since this is a multiple choice question, instead of doing algebra we'll just plug in the choices and find the one that works. The only one that works is choice B, so that $p_A = 150$ torr, $p_B = 75$ torr, and $p_C = 75$ torr, for a total of 300 torr.

Example 8-14: If the ratio of the partial pressures of a pair of gases mixed together in a sealed vessel is 3:1 at 300 K, what would be the ratio of their partial pressures at 400 K?

A) 3:1
B) 4:1
C) 4:3
D) 12:1

Solution: Remember that the partial pressure of a gas is the way that we talk about the amount of gas in a mixture. The question states that the ratio of partial pressures of two gases is 3:1. That just means there's three times more of one than the other. Regardless of the temperature, if the vessel is sealed, then there will always be three times more of one than the other. Choice A is the correct answer.

8.5 GRAHAM'S LAW OF EFFUSION

The escape of a gas molecule through a very tiny hole (comparable in size to the molecules themselves) into an evacuated region is called **effusion**:

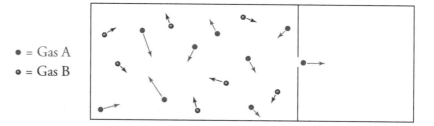

● = Gas A
○ = Gas B

The gases in the left-hand container are at the same temperature, so their average kinetic energies are the same. If Gas A and Gas B have different molar masses, the heavier molecules will move, on average, slower than the lighter ones will. We can be even more precise. The average kinetic energy of a molecule of Gas A is $\frac{1}{2}m_A(v_A^2)_{avg}$, and the average kinetic energy of a molecule of Gas B is $\frac{1}{2}m_B(v_B^2)_{avg}$. Setting these equal to each other, we get

$$\frac{1}{2}m_A(v_A^2)_{avg} = \frac{1}{2}m_B(v_B^2)_{avg} \quad \Rightarrow \quad \frac{(v_A^2)_{avg}}{(v_B^2)_{avg}} = \frac{m_B}{m_A} \quad \Rightarrow \quad \frac{\text{rms } v_A}{\text{rms } v_B} = \sqrt{\frac{m_B}{m_A}}$$

(The abbreviation **rms** stands for *root-mean-square*; it's the square root of the mean [average] of the square of speed. Therefore, rms v is a convenient measure of the average speed of the molecules.) For example, if Gas A is hydrogen gas (H_2, molecular weight = 2) and Gas B is oxygen gas (O_2, molecular weight = 32), the hydrogen molecules will move, on average,

$$\sqrt{\frac{m_B}{m_A}} = \sqrt{\frac{32}{2}} = \sqrt{16} = 4$$

times faster than the oxygen molecules.

This result—which follows from one of the assumptions of the kinetic-molecular theory (namely that the average kinetic energy of the molecules of a gas is proportional to the temperature)—can be confirmed experimentally by performing an effusion experiment. Which gas should escape faster? The rate at which a gas effuses should depend directly on how fast its molecules move; the faster they travel, the more often they'd "collide" with the hole and escape. So we'd expect that if we compared the effusion rates for Gases A and B, we'd get a ratio equal to the ratio of their average speeds (if the molecules of Gas A travel 4 times faster than those of Gas B, then Gas A should effuse 4 times faster). Since we just figured out that the ratio of their average speeds is equal to the reciprocal of the square root of the ratio of their masses, we'd expect the ratio of their effusion rates to be the same. This result is known as **Graham's law of effusion**:

Graham's Law of Effusion

$$\frac{\text{rate of effusion of Gas A}}{\text{rate of effusion of Gas B}} = \sqrt{\frac{\text{molar mass of Gas B}}{\text{molar mass of Gas A}}}$$

Let's emphasize the distinction between the relationships of temperature to the kinetic energy and to the speed of the gas. The molecules of two different gases at the same temperature have the same average kinetic energy. But the molecules of two different gases at the same temperature don't have the same average *speed*. Lighter molecules travel faster, because the kinetic energy depends on both the mass and the speed of the molecules.

Also, it's important to remember that not all the molecules of the gas in a container—even if there's only one type of molecule—travel at the same speed. Their speeds cover a wide range. What we *can* say is that as the temperature of the sample is increased, the *average* speed increases. In fact, since $KE \propto T$, the root-mean-square speed is proportional to $\sqrt{T}$. The figure below shows the distribution of molecular speeds for a gas at three different temperatures. Notice that the rms speeds increase as the temperature is increased.

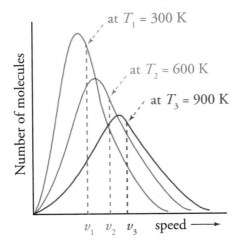

Example 8-15: A container holds methane (CH_4) and sulfur dioxide (SO_2), at a temperature of 227°C. Let v_M denote the rms speed of the methane molecules and v_S the rms speed of the sulfur dioxide molecules. Which of the following best describes the relationship between these speeds?

A) $v_S = 16\, v_M$
B) $v_S = 2\, v_M$
C) $v_M = 2\, v_S$
D) $v_M = 16\, v_S$

Solution: The molecular weight of methane is $12 + 4(1) = 16$, and the molecular weight of sulfur dioxide is $32 + 2(16) = 64$. Therefore

$$\frac{v_M}{v_S} = \sqrt{\frac{m_S}{m_M}} = \sqrt{\frac{64}{16}} = \sqrt{4} = 2 \quad \Rightarrow \quad v_M = 2v_S$$

So, choice C is the answer.

Example 8-16: In a laboratory experiment, Chamber A holds a mixture of four gases: 1 mole each of chlorine, fluorine, nitrogen, and carbon dioxide. A tiny hole is made in the side of the chamber, and the gases are allowed to effuse from Chamber A into an empty container. When 2 moles of gas have escaped, which gas will have the greatest mole fraction in Chamber A?

A) $Cl_2(g)$
B) $F_2(g)$
C) $N_2(g)$
D) $CO_2(g)$

Solution: The gas with the greatest mole fraction remaining in Chamber A will be the gas with the *slowest* rate of effusion. This is the gas with the highest molecular weight. Of the gases in the chamber, Cl_2 has the greatest molecular weight. Therefore, the answer is A.

Example 8-17: A balloon holds a mixture of fluorine, $F_2(g)$, and helium, $He(g)$. If the rms speed of helium atoms is 540 m/s, what is the rms speed of the fluorine molecules?

Solution: The molecular weight of F_2 is $2(19) = 38$, and the molecular weight of He is 4. Therefore,

$$\frac{v_{F_2}}{v_{He}} = \sqrt{\frac{m_{He}}{m_{F_2}}} = \sqrt{\frac{4}{38}} \approx \sqrt{\frac{1}{9}} = \frac{1}{3} \quad \Rightarrow \quad v_{F_2} \approx \frac{1}{3}v_{He} = \frac{1}{3}(540 \text{ m/s}) = 180 \text{ m/s}$$

Example 8-18: A container holds methane (CH_4) and sulfur dioxide (SO_2) at a temperature of 227°C. Let KE_M denote the average kinetic energy of the methane molecules and KE_S the average kinetic energy of the sulfur dioxide molecules. Which of the following best describes the relationship between these energies?

A) $KE_S = 4\, KE_M$
B) $KE_S = 3\, KE_M$
C) $KE_M = KE_S$
D) $KE_M = 4\, KE_S$

Solution: Since both gases are at the same temperature, the average kinetic energies of their molecules will be the *same* (remember: $KE_{avg} \propto T$). Thus, the answer is C.

Example 8-19: The temperature of neon gas in a glass tube is increased from 10°C to 160°C. As a result, the average kinetic energy of the neon atoms will increase by a factor of:

A) less than 2.
B) 2.
C) 4.
D) 16.

8.5

Solution: We use the fact that $KE_{avg} \propto T$. However, don't fall for the trap of thinking that the temperature has increased by a factor of 16. Calculations involving the gas laws (and that includes the proportionality between KE_{avg} and T from kinetic-molecular theory) must be done with temperatures expressed in *kelvins*. The temperature here increased from 283 K to 433 K, which is less than a factor of 2 increase. Therefore, KE_{avg} will also increase by a factor of less than 2 (choice A).

Chapter 8 Summary

- The pressure of a gas is due to the collisions gas particles have with the container walls.

- The ideal gas law states that $PV = nRT$.

- Standard temperature and pressure (STP) conditions are at 1 atm and 273 K. Under these conditions, 1 mol of any gas will occupy 22.4 L of space.

- Particles of an ideal gas take up no volume and experience no intermolecular forces. They also have elastic collisions with each other and the walls of their container.

- Real gases approach ideal behavior under most conditions, but deviate most from ideal behavior under conditions of high pressure and low temperature.

- Real gases can be quantified using the van der Waals equation:

$$\left(P + \frac{an^2}{V^2}\right)(V - nb) = nRT$$

- Dalton's law of partial pressures states that the total pressure inside a container is equal to the sum of the partial pressures of each constituent gas. The partial pressure of a gas divided by the total pressure of all gases is equal to its mole fraction within the gaseous mixture.

- Temperature is a measure of the average kinetic energy of molecules within a sample.

- Graham's law of effusion states that the rate of effusion of a gas is inversely proportional to its molecular weight. In other words, lighter gases effuse more quickly than heavier gases.

CHAPTER 8 FREESTANDING PRACTICE QUESTIONS

1. A sample of nitrogen gas is heated in a sealed, rigid container. The pressure inside the container increases because the added energy causes:

A) some of the nitrogen molecules to split, so more particles contribute to increase the pressure.
B) the molecules of gas to move faster, increasing the frequency of intermolecular collisions.
C) the molecules of gas to move faster, increasing the frequency of collisions with the container.
D) the molecules of gas to stick together in clusters that have a greater momentum.

2. Two identical balloons are filled with different gases at STP. Balloon A contains 0.25 moles of neon, and balloon B contains 0.25 moles of oxygen. Which of the following properties would be greater for balloon B?

A) Density
B) Volume
C) Number of particles
D) Average kinetic energy

3. The figure below depicts the relative sizes and mole fractions of two monatomic gases in a closed container.

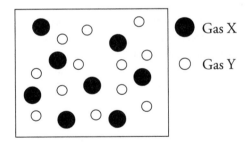

Which of the following is true about the gas mixture after a small hole is punched in the container and the gases are allowed to completely effuse?

A) The partial pressure of Gas X will never equal the partial pressure of Gas Y.
B) The partial pressure of Gas Y will decrease faster than the partial pressure of Gas X.
C) The partial pressure of Gas Y will increase because the mole fraction of Gas Y will increase.
D) The partial pressures of each gas will remain unchanged.

4. There are an unknown number of moles of argon in a steel container. A chemist injects two moles of nitrogen into the container. The temperature and volume do not change, but the pressure increases by ten percent. Originally the container held:

A) 16 moles of Ar.
B) 18 moles of Ar.
C) 20 moles of Ar.
D) 22 moles of Ar.

5. Which of the following gases will deviate most from ideal behavior?

A) NO_2
B) CO_2
C) CS_2
D) N_2O

6. Which of the following is true for a closed flask containing both 1 mole of ideal Gas X and 1 mole of real Gas Y?

A) The total energy of X is equal to the total energy of Y.
B) The average kinetic energy of X is equal to the average kinetic energy of Y.
C) The total volume available to the gases is the same as the total volume of the flask.
D) Gases X and Y are at different temperatures.

7. Given the following combustion reaction, calculate the mole fraction of hydrocarbon in the reactant solution before combustion. Assume neither starting material is limiting.

$$Z\ C_xH_y(g) + 8\ O_2(g) \rightarrow 5\ CO_2(g) + 6\ H_2O(l)$$

A) 1/8
B) 1/9
C) 2/9
D) 1/3

CHAPTER 8 PRACTICE PASSAGE

As a part of ongoing human metabolism, oxygen combines with fuels to yield ATP, CO_2, and H_2O. Hence the tissues tend constantly to reduce the blood's oxygen concentration and increase its carbon dioxide concentration. The lungs serve to replenish the blood's oxygen supply and to empty it of accumulated carbon dioxide via the process of passive diffusion. The lungs are also the delivery organ for gas phase pharmacological agents, the absorption of which is a characteristic trait of the specific drug compound.

During inspiration, contraction of the diaphragm produces negative pressure change in the lungs, and air therefore moves from the atmosphere into the lungs. At the level of the alveoli, carbon dioxide continuously moves from capillary blood into the lungs, and oxygen moves from the lungs into the blood. The net result is that the partial pressure of oxygen in the lungs is 100 torr, which is 59 torr less than the partial pressure of oxygen in the atmosphere. Partial pressure of carbon dioxide in the lungs is 40 torr greater than in the atmosphere.

The total pressure of gases in the lungs is the sum of the partial pressures of each of the individual gases. Equation 1 below shows the result of substituting values for partial pressures into the ideal gas law equation. P_t represents the total pressure of the gases, and the n's denote the numbers of moles of the individual, nonreactive gases. As air passes from the atmosphere to the alveoli, the partial pressures of both nitrogen and oxygen decrease (although nitrogen is not absorbed by the alveoli to any appreciable extent).

$$P_t = (n_1 + n_2 + n_3 + \ldots)RT/V$$

Equation 1

Gas	Pressure (torr)		
	Atmosphere	Inspired air	Alveolar air
N_2	595	564	573
O_2	159	149	100
H_2O	6	47	47
CO_2	0	0	40

Table 1

Inhaled bioactive compounds, such as anesthetics, must be present in concentrations sufficient for the absorption of a biologically relevant concentration, but not so much that large amounts of the compounds are exhaled and wasted. The alveolar concentration of a particular anesthetic required to prevent movement (motor response) in response to surgical (pain) stimulus is known as the compound's MAC (minimum alveolar concentration).

1. Which of the following causes the exchange of oxygen and carbon dioxide between the lungs and bloodstream?

A) Concentration gradients
B) Different values for the gas constant
C) Greater permeability of oxygen
D) Decreased volumes of gases in the bloodstream

2. Between the time it is inhaled from the atmosphere and the time it is exhaled, air experiences a greater decrease in molar quantity of which gas: oxygen or nitrogen?

A) Oxygen, because nitrogen is less reactive than oxygen in the gaseous state.
B) Oxygen, because it diffuses from lung to capillary.
C) Nitrogen, because nitrogen is not soluble in the bloodstream.
D) Nitrogen, because the proportionally lesser partial pressure decrease corresponds to a proportionally greater decrease in molar quantity.

3. The relationship between the partial pressure of a gas (P) and the number of moles of that gas (n) is best represented by which of the following graphs?

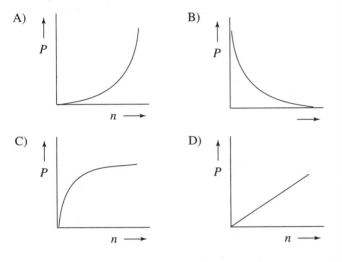

A)

B)

C)

D)

4. Which one of the following expressions can be used to compare atmospheric air and alveolar air and calculate the reduction in the number of moles of oxygen present in the alveoli?

A) $(V/RT)(100)$
B) $(V/RT)(149 – 100)$
C) $(V/RT)(159 – 100)$
D) $(V/RT)(159 – 149)$

5. If the MAC of the anesthetic Sevoflurane is 2.1 vol%, what is the partial pressure of Sevoflurane that must be maintained in the alveoli to ensure anesthetic potency?

A) 16 torr
B) 32 torr
C) 87 torr
D) 160 torr

SOLUTIONS TO CHAPTER 8 FREESTANDING PRACTICE QUESTIONS

1. **C** According to kinetic molecular theory, pressure is defined by the frequency of collisions between gas particles and the walls of their container. While increasing the temperature of the gas will cause more collisions between particles as well, these collisions do not define pressure (eliminate choice B). In addition, collisions between particles are elastic, so unless the particles are highly polar and have a strong attraction for each other (the gas is behaving non-ideally), they will not stick together. Since N_2 is non-polar it should behave ideally, so choice D can be eliminated. Finally, nitrogen is a very stable diatomic element, and heating a sample of nitrogen is not likely to break the strong triple bond between nitrogen atoms, eliminating choice A.

2. **A** Since both balloons contain the same number of moles of gas under identical pressure and temperature conditions (STP), they should have the same volume (in this case 5.6 L since 1 mol = 22.4 L). Eliminate choice B. An identical amount of each gas is added to each balloon, so they should also contain the same number of gas particles (0.25 mol × 6.02 × 10²³ particles/mol), eliminating choice C. Since the gases are at the same temperature they will have the same average kinetic energy, so by process of elimination, A must be the correct answer. Density is mass/volume. Since the two gases have the same volume, oxygen, with a larger molar mass (O_2 = 32 g/mol vs. Ne = 20 g/mol), will have the greater density.

3. **B** After a hole is punched in the container and the gases begin to escape, the total pressure of the container will decrease, and the individual partial pressures of the gases will therefore also decrease. Eliminate choices C and D. According to Graham's law, the lighter the gas molecule, the faster its rate of effusion through a small hole. Gas Y will effuse faster than Gas X, so its partial pressure will decrease at a faster rate. The gases are allowed to completely effuse and the figure indicates that the mole fraction of Y is slightly larger than X. Therefore there will most likely be a moment in time when the partial pressures of both gases are equal (and this will definitely be the case when the container is finally empty), eliminating choice A.

4. **C** At constant V and T, the pressure of an ideal gas reflects the number of particles (regardless of their identity). It is a simplification of the ideal gas law from $PV = nRT$ to $P \propto n$. So, if the addition of two moles of N_2 into the chamber results in an increase in P of 10 percent, then the moles added must be 10 percent of the initial number of Ar moles. Two moles are 10 percent of 20 moles.

5. **C** The most ideal gases are those that have the smallest molecular volumes and the weakest intermolecular forces. The compounds in choices A, B, and D are made of elements in the second period, making them very similar in size, whereas CS_2 (choice C) has two sulfur atoms which are in the third period. Carbon disulfide therefore has a significantly larger molecular volume than the others, and relatively strong London dispersion forces as a result. Choice C therefore deviates the most from ideal behavior.

6. **B** Temperature is a measure of average kinetic energy. If gases X and Y are in the same flask they must be at the same temperature, eliminating choice D and making choice B correct. The total energy of a gas is equal to its kinetic energy plus its potential energy. Since Gas Y is a real gas and experiences intermolecular forces, it has potential energy, whereas ideal Gas X does not. Therefore, choice A is eliminated. Real gas molecules occupy some volume in the container, whereas ideal gases have no molecular volume. Since the flask contains a real gas, the total volume available to the gases is slightly less than the total volume of the flask, eliminating choice C.

7. **B** First, balance the equation:

$$C_5H_{12}(g) + 8\ O_2(g) \rightarrow 5\ CO_2(g) + 6\ H_2O(l)$$

The hydrocarbon must be C_5H_{12} and the coefficient Z is 1. Since the question indicates that neither reactant is limiting, there must be a 1:8 molar ratio of hydrocarbon to oxygen present in the reaction flask, so the mole fraction (X) of hydrocarbon in the reactant solution before combustion is calculated by:

$$X = \text{(moles hydrocarbon)/(total moles)}$$

$$X = 1/(1+8) = 1/9$$

SOLUTIONS TO CHAPTER 8 PRACTICE PASSAGE

1. **A** The passage states that gases move by passive diffusion. Molecules undergo passive diffusion due to concentration gradients (they diffuse from high to low concentrations).

2. **B** According to the data in Table 1, oxygen experiences the greater decrease in partial pressure (this eliminates choices C and D). This drop is due to the binding of oxygen to hemoglobin in the capillaries.

3. **D** Partial pressure is proportional to the number of moles of the gas. The graph of a proportion is a straight line through the origin: the graph in choice D.

4. **C** Since $n = (V/RT)P$, we have $\Delta n = (V/RT)\Delta P = (V/RT)(159\ \text{torr} - 100\ \text{torr})$ from Table 1.

5. **A** The overall pressure in the alveoli must be equal to atmospheric pressure (760 torr), which is confirmed by summing the values in Table 1. Assuming at least a rough ideal gas behavior, a volume percentage is equivalent to a molar percentage and therefore the percentage of partial pressure associated with it by Equation 1. The pressure representing 2.1% of 760 torr can be quickly ascertained by realizing that 1% is 7.6 torr, meaning 2% is 15.2 torr. As such, 2.1% is roughly 16 torr.

Chapter 9
Kinetics

9.1 REACTION MECHANISM: AN ANALOGY

Chemical **kinetics** is the study of how reactions take place and how fast they occur. (Kinetics tells us nothing about the *spontaneity* of a reaction, however!)

Consider this scenario: A group of people are washing a pile of dirty dishes and stacking them up as clean, dry dishes. Our "reaction" has dirty dishes as starting material, and clean, dry dishes as the product:

$$\text{dirty dish} \rightarrow \text{clean-and-dry dish}$$

But what about a *soapy* dish? We know it's part of the process, but the equation doesn't include it. When we break down the pathway of a dirty dish to a clean-and-dry dish, we realize that the reaction happens in several steps, a sequence of **elementary** steps that show us the reaction **mechanism:**

1) dirty dish $\rightarrow$ soapy dish
2) soapy dish $\rightarrow$ rinsed dish
3) rinsed dish $\rightarrow$ clean-and-dry dish

The soapy and rinsed dishes are reaction **intermediates**. They are necessary for the conversion of dirty dishes to clean-and-dry dishes, but don't appear either in the starting material or products. If you add up all the reactants and products, the intermediates cancel out, and you'll have the overall equation.

In the same way, we write chemical reactions as if they occur in a single step:

$$2\,NO + O_2 \rightarrow 2\,NO_2$$

But in reality, things are a little more complicated, and reactions often proceed through intermediates that we don't show in the chemical equation. The truth for the reaction above is that it occurs in two steps:

1) $2\,NO \rightarrow N_2O_2$
2) $N_2O_2 + O_2 \rightarrow 2\,NO_2$

The N_2O_2 comes and goes during the reaction, but isn't part of the starting material or products. N_2O_2 is a reaction intermediate.

Just as the soapy dishes and rinsed dishes are produced and then consumed, we can identify an **intermediate** in a series of elementary steps as a substance that is produced in one elementary step and then consumed in a subsequent step. Although the two elementary steps don't need to be sequential, they often are. As above, note that intermediates will not be part of the overall balanced chemical reaction. Depending on the rate of the elementary step that consumes the intermediate, the concentration of the intermediate will vary in solution. As the consuming elementary step becomes faster, the steady-state concentration of the intermediate becomes smaller, and it becomes harder to detect the intermediate.

Rate-Determining Step

What determines the rate of a reaction? Consider our friends doing the dishes.

1) dirty dish → soapy dish   Bingo washes at 5 dishes per minute.

2) soapy dish → rinsed dish   Ringo rinses at 8 dishes per minute.

3) rinsed dish → clean-and-dry dish   Dingo dries at 3 dishes per minute.

What will be the rate of the overall reaction? Thanks to Dingo, the dishes move from dirty to clean-and-dry at only 3 dishes a minute. It doesn't matter how fast Bingo and Ringo wash and rinse; the dishes will pile up behind Dingo. The **rate-determining step** is Dingo's drying step, and true to its name, it determines the overall rate of reaction.

The slowest step in a process determines the overall reaction rate.

This applies to chemical reactions as well. For our chemical reaction given above, we have

$$2 \text{ NO} \rightarrow \text{N}_2\text{O}_2 \quad \text{(fast)}$$

$$\text{N}_2\text{O}_2 + \text{O}_2 \rightarrow 2 \text{ NO}_2 \quad \text{(slow)}$$

The second step is the slowest, and it will determine the overall rate of reaction. No matter how fast the first step moves along, the intermediates will pile up in front of the second step as it plods along. The slow step dictates the rate of the overall reaction.

Once again, there's an important difference between our dishes analogy and a chemical reaction: While the dishes pile up behind Dingo, in a chemical reaction the intermediates will not pile up. Rather they will shuttle back and forth between reactants and products until the slow step takes it forward. This would be like taking a rinsed dish and getting it soapy again, until Dingo is ready for it!

Example 9-1: Which of the following is the best example of a rate?

A)   rate = $\Delta[A]/\Delta t$
B)   rate = $\Delta[A]/\Delta[B]$
C)   rate = $\Delta[A]\Delta[B]$
D)   rate = $\Delta[A]^2$

Solution: Regardless of the topic, rate is always defined as change in something over change in time. Choice A is the answer.

9.2 REACTION RATE

The **rate** of a reaction indicates how fast reactants are being consumed or how fast products are being formed. The reaction rate depends on several factors. Since the reactant molecules must collide and interact in order for old bonds to be broken and new ones to be formed to generate the product molecules, anything that affects these collisions and interactions will affect the reaction rate. The reaction rate is determined by the following:

1) How frequently the reactant molecules collide
2) The orientation of the colliding molecules
3) Their energy

Activation Energy

Every chemical reaction has an **activation energy** (E_a), or the minimum energy required of reactant molecules during a molecular collision in order for the reaction to proceed to products. If the reactant molecules don't possess this much energy, their collisions won't be able to produce the products and the reaction will not occur. If the reactants possess the necessary activation energy, they can reach a high-energy (and short-lived!) **transition state**, also known as the **activated complex**. For example, if the reaction is $A_2 + B_2 \rightarrow 2\,AB$, say, the activated complex might look something like this:

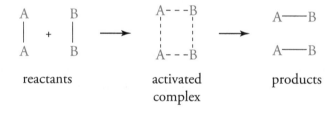

| reactants | activated complex | products |

Now that we have introduced all species that might appear throughout the course of a chemical reaction, we can illustrate the energy changes that occur as a reaction occurs in a **reaction coordinate diagram**. Consider the following two-step process and its reaction coordinate graph below:

$$\text{Step 1:} \quad A \rightarrow X$$
$$\text{Step 2:} \quad X \rightarrow B$$
$$\overline{\text{Overall reaction:} \quad A \rightarrow B}$$

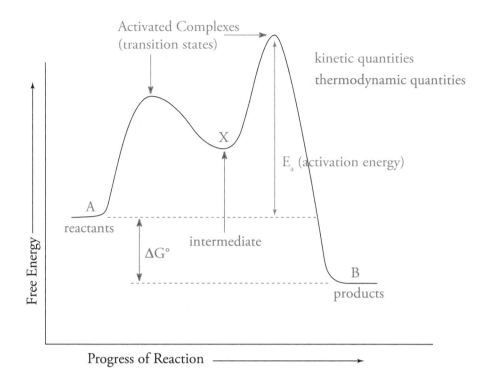

Notice that the transition state is always an energy maximum, and is therefore distinct from an intermediate. Remember that reaction intermediates (shown as X in this case) are produced in an early step of the mechanism, and are later used up so they do not appear as products of the overall reaction. The intermediate is shown here as a local minimum in terms of its energy, but has more energy than either the reactants or products. The high energy intermediate is therefore highly reactive, making it difficult to isolate.

Since the progress of the reaction depends on the reactant molecules colliding with enough energy to generate the activated complex, we can make the following statements concerning the reaction rate:

1) *The lower the activation energy, the faster the reaction rate.* The reaction coordinate above suggests that the second step of the mechanism will therefore be the slow step, or the rate-determining step, since the second "hill" of the diagram is higher.

2) *The greater the concentrations of the reactants, the faster the reaction rate.* Favorable collisions are more likely as the concentrations of reactant molecules increase.

3) *The higher the temperature of the reaction mixture, the faster the reaction rate.* At higher temperatures, more reactant molecules have a sufficient energy to overcome the activation-energy barrier, and molecules collide at a higher frequency, so the reaction can proceed at a faster rate.

Notice in the reaction coordinate diagram above that the $\Delta G°$ of the reaction has no bearing on the rate of the reaction, and vice versa. Thermodynamic factors and kinetic factors *do not affect each other* (a concept the MCAT loves to ask about).

9.3 CATALYSTS

Catalysts provide reactants with a different route, usually a shortcut, to get to products. A **catalyst** will almost always make a reaction go faster by either speeding up the rate-determining step or providing an optimized route to products. A catalyst that accelerates a reaction does so *by lowering the activation energy* of the rate-determining step, and therefore the energy of the highest-energy transition state:

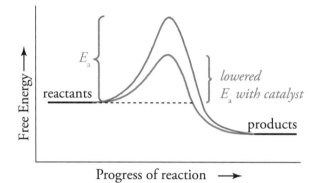

The key difference between a reactant and a catalyst is that the reactants are converted to products, but *a catalyst remains unchanged at the end of a reaction*. A catalyst can undergo a temporary change during a reaction, but it is always converted back to its original state. Like reaction intermediates, catalysts aren't included in the overall reaction equation.

Our dish crew could use a catalyst. Picture Dingo walking to pick up each wet dish, drying it on both sides, and walking back to place it in the clean dish stack. Now imagine a helper, Daisy, who takes the wet dish from Ringo, then walks it over to Dingo, and while he dries and stacks, she returns with another wet dish. This way, Dingo can dry 5 dishes a minute instead of 3, and the overall dish-cleaning rate increases to 5 dishes a minute. Daisy is the catalyst, but the chain of events in the overall reaction remains the same.

In the same way, chemical reactions can be catalyzed. Consider the decomposition of ozone:

$$O_3(g) + O(g) \rightarrow 2\ O_2(g)$$

This reaction actually takes place in two steps and is catalyzed by nitric oxide (NO):

1) $NO(g) + O_3(g) \rightarrow NO_2(g) + O_2(g)$
2) $NO_2(g) + O(g) \rightarrow NO(g) + O_2(g)$

NO(g) is necessary for this reaction to proceed at a noticeable rate, and even undergoes changes itself during the process. But NO(g) remains unchanged at the end of the reaction and makes the reaction occur much faster than it would in its absence. NO(g), a product of automobile exhaust, is a catalyst in ozone destruction.

It is important to note that the addition of a catalyst will affect the rate of a reaction, but not the equilibrium or the thermodynamics of the reaction. A catalyst provides a different pathway for the reactants to get to the products, and lowers the activation energy, E_a. But a catalyst does not change any of the thermodynamic quantities such as ΔG, ΔH, and ΔS of a reaction.

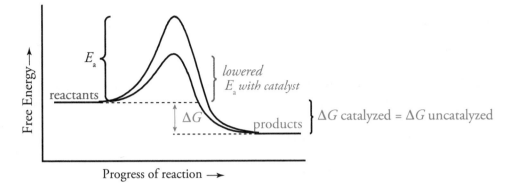

Example 9-2: Which of the following statements is true?

A) Catalysts decrease the activation energy of the forward reaction only.
B) Catalysts decrease the activation energy of the reverse reaction only.
C) Catalysts decrease the activation energy of both the forward and reverse reactions.
D) Catalysts decrease the activation energy of the forward reaction and increase the activation energy of the reverse reaction.

Solution: Catalysts decrease the activation energy of the forward reaction and reverse reaction—that's why they have no net effect on a system that's already at equilibrium. Choice C is the correct choice.

Example 9-3: Which of the following is true about the hypothetical two-step reaction shown below?

1) $A + 2B \rightarrow C + 2D$ (fast)
2) $C \rightarrow A + E$ (slow)

A) A is a catalyst, and C is an intermediate.
B) A is a catalyst, and D is an intermediate.
C) B is a catalyst, and A is an intermediate.
D) B is a catalyst, and C is an intermediate.

Solution: C is an intermediate; it's formed in one step and consumed in the other. This eliminates choices B and C. Now, is A or B the catalyst? Notice that B is consumed but not reformed; therefore, it cannot be the catalyst. The answer is A.

Example 9-4: A reaction is run without a catalyst and is found to have an activation energy of 140 kJ/mol and a heat of reaction, ΔH, of 30 kJ/mol. In the presence of a catalyst, however, the activation energy is reduced to 120 kJ/mol. What will be the heat of reaction in the presence of the catalyst?

A) –10 kJ/mol
B) 10 kJ/mol
C) 30 kJ/mol
D) 50 kJ/mol

Solution: Catalysts affect only the kinetics of a reaction, not the thermodynamics. The heat of the reaction will be the same with or without a catalyst. The answer is C.

9.4 RATE LAWS

On the MCAT, you might be given data about the rate of a particular reaction and be asked to derive the **rate law**. The data for rate laws are determined by the *initial rates* of reaction and typically are given as the **rate at which the reactant disappears**. You'll rarely see products in a rate law expression, usually only reactants. What does a rate law tell us? Although a reaction needs all the reactants to proceed, *only those that are involved in the rate-determining step (the slow step) are part of the rate law expression*. Some reactants may not affect the reaction rate at all, and so they won't be a part of the rate law expression.

Let's look at a generic reaction, $a\,A + b\,B \rightarrow c\,C + d\,D$, and its rate law:

$$\text{rate} = k[A]^x[B]^y$$

where

$$x = \text{the \textbf{order} of the reaction with respect to A}$$

$$y = \text{the \textbf{order} of the reaction with respect to B}$$

$$(x + y) = \text{the \textbf{overall order} of the reaction}$$

$$k = \text{the rate constant}$$

The rate law can only be determined *experimentally*. You *can't* get the orders of the reactants, not to mention the rate constant k, just by looking at the balanced equation. The exception to this rule is for an *elementary step* in a reaction mechanism. The rate law is first order for a unimolecular elementary step and second order for a **bimolecular** elementary step. The individual order of the reactants in a rate law will follow from their stoichiometry in the rate-determining step (similar to the way they're included in an equilibrium constant).

Let's look at a set of reaction rate data and see how to determine the rate law for the reaction

$$A + B + C \rightarrow D + E$$

Experiment	[A]	[B]	[C]	Initial reaction rate [M/s]
1	0.2 M	0.1 M	0.05 M	1×10^{-3}
2	0.4 M	0.1 M	0.05 M	2×10^{-3}
3	0.2 M	0.2 M	0.05 M	4×10^{-3}
4	0.2 M	0.1 M	0.10 M	1×10^{-3}

From the experimental data, we can determine the orders with respect to the reactants—that is, the exponents x, y, and z in the equation

$$\text{rate} = k[A]^x[B]^y[C]^z$$

and the overall order of the reaction, $x + y + z$.

Let's first find the order of the reaction with respect to Reactant A. As we go from Experiment 1 to Experiment 2, only [A] changes, so we can use the data to figure out the order of the reaction with respect to Reactant [A]. We notice that the value of [A] doubled, and the reaction rate doubled. Therefore, the reaction rate is proportional to [A], and $x = 1$.

Next, let's look at [B]. As we go from Experiment 1 to Experiment 3, only [B] changes. When [B] is doubled, the rate is quadrupled. Therefore, the rate is proportional to $[B]^2$, and $y = 2$.

Finally, let's look at [C]. As we go from Experiment 1 to Experiment 4, only [C] changes. When [C] is doubled, the rate is unaffected. This tells us that the reaction rate does not depend on [C], so $z = 0$.

Therefore, the rate law has the form

$$\text{rate} = k[A][B]^2$$

The reaction is first order with respect to [A], second order with respect to [B], zero order with respect to [C], and third order overall. In general, if a reaction rate increases by a factor f when the concentration of a reactant increases by a factor c, and $f = c^x$, then we can say that x is the order with respect to that reactant.

The Rate Constant

From the experimental data, you can also calculate the rate constant, k. For the reaction we looked at above, we found that the rate law is given by: rate $= k[A][B]^2$. Solving this for k, we get

$$k = \frac{\text{rate}}{[A][B]^2}$$

Now, just pick any experiment in the table, and using the results of Experiment 1, you'd find that

$$k = \frac{\text{rate}}{[A][B]^2} = \frac{1 \times 10^{-3}}{(0.2)(0.1)^2} = 0.5$$

Any of the experiments will give you the same value for k because it's a constant for any given reaction at a given temperature. That is, each reaction has its own rate constant, which takes into account such factors as the frequency of collisions, the fraction of the collisions with the proper orientation to initiate the desired bond changes, and the activation energy. This can be expressed mathematically with the **Arrhenius equation**:

$$k = Ae^{-(E_a/RT)}$$

Here, A is the Arrhenius factor (which takes into account the orientation of the colliding molecules), E_a is the activation energy, R is the gas-law constant, and T is the temperature in kelvins. If we rewrite this equation in the form $\ln k = \ln A - (E_a/RT)$, we can more clearly see that *adding a catalyst* (thus decreasing

E_a) or *increasing the temperature* will increase k. In either case, the expression E_a/RT decreases, and subtracting something smaller gives a greater result, so ln k (and thus k itself) will increase. (By the way, a rough rule of thumb is that the rate will increase by a factor of about 2 to 4 for every 10-degree (Celsius) increase in temperature.)

The units of the rate constant are not necessarily uniform from one reaction to the next. Reactions of different orders will have rate constants bearing different units. In order to obtain the units of the rate constant one must keep in mind that the rate, on the left side of the equation, must always have units of M/s as it measures the change in concentration of a species in the reaction over time. The units given to the rate constant must, when combined with the units of the concentrations in the rate equation, provide M/s.

Below is a generic second order rate equation.

$$\text{Rate} = k[A][B]$$

Assuming that the concentrations of both A and B are in molarity (M), then in order to give the left side of the equation units of M/s, the units of the rate constant must be $M^{-1}s^{-1}$. If the rate were third order, the units would be $M^{-2}s^{-1}$, or if first order then simply s^{-1}.

Experiment	[A]	[B]	Initial reaction rate [M/s]
1	0.01 M	0.01 M	4.0×10^{-3}
2	0.01 M	0.02 M	8.0×10^{-3}
3	0.02 M	0.02 M	1.6×10^{-2}
4	0.04 M	0.02 M	3.2×10^{-2}

Example 9-5: Based on the data given above, determine the rate law for the reaction A + B → C.

A) Rate = $k[B]$
B) Rate = $k[A][B]$
C) Rate = $k[A]^2[B]$
D) Rate = $k[A][B]^2$

Solution: Comparing Experiments 1 and 2, we notice that when [B] doubled (and [A] remained unchanged), the reaction rate doubled. Therefore, the reaction is first order with respect to [B]; this eliminates choice D. Now, comparing Experiments 3 and 4, we notice that when [A] doubled (and [B] remained unchanged), the reaction rate also doubled. This means that the reaction is first order with respect to [A] as well. Therefore, the answer is B.

Example 9-6: Which of the following gives the form of the rate law for the balanced reaction

$$4\,A + 2\,B \;\rightarrow\; C + 3\,D?$$

A)   Rate = $k[A]^4[B]^2$
B)   Rate = $k[A]^2[B]$
C)   Rate = $k[C][D]^3/[A]^4[B]^2$
D)   Cannot be determined from the information given

Solution: Unless the given reaction is the rate-determining, elementary step, we have no way of knowing what the rate law is. The answer is D.

Experiment	[A]	[B]	Initial reaction rate [M/s]
1	0.1 M	0.2 M	2.0×10^{-5}
2	0.2 M	0.3 M	1.2×10^{-4}
3	0.1 M	0.4 M	4.0×10^{-5}
4	0.2 M	0.4 M	1.6×10^{-4}

Example 9-7: Using the data given above, determine the numerical value of the rate constant for the reaction $A + B \rightarrow C$.

Solution: First, let's find the rate law. Comparing Experiments 3 and 4, we notice that when [A] doubled (and [B] remained unchanged), the reaction rate increased by a factor of 4. This means the reaction is second order with respect to [A]. Comparing Experiments 1 and 3, we notice that when [B] doubled (and [A] remained unchanged), the reaction rate increased by a factor of 2. This means the reaction is first order with respect to [B]. Therefore, the rate law is *rate* = $k[A]^2[B]$. Finally, using any of the experiments, we can solve for k; using the data in Experiment 1, say, we find that

$$k = \frac{\text{rate}}{[A]^2[B]} = \frac{2 \times 10^{-5}\,M/s}{2 \times 10^{-3}\,M^3} = 10^{-2}\,M^{-2}\,s^{-1} = 0.01\,M^{-2}\,s^{-1}$$

Chapter 9 Summary

· Kinetics is the study of how quickly a reaction occurs, but does not determine *whether or not* a reaction will occur.

· All rates are experimentally determined by measuring a change in the concentration of a reactant or product compared to a change in time (often given in *M*/s).

· Molecules must collide in order to react, and the frequency and energy of these collisions determines how fast the reaction occurs.

· Increasing the concentration of reactants *often* increases the reaction rate due to an increased number of collisions.

· Increasing the temperature of a reaction *always* increases the reaction rate since molecules move faster and collide more frequently; the energy of collisions also increases.

· Activation energy (E_a) is the minimum energy required to start a reaction and decreases in the presence of a catalyst, thereby increasing the reaction rate.

· Transition states are at energy maxima, while intermediates are at local energy minima along a reaction coordinate.

· A reaction mechanism must agree with experimental data, and suggests a possible pathway by which reactants and intermediates might collide in order for a chemical reaction to occur.

· The sum of all elementary steps of a mechanism will add to give the overall chemical reaction.

· The slow step of the mechanism is the rate limiting step, and determines the rate of the overall reaction.

· A rate law can only be determined from experimental data or if given a mechanism, and has the general form: Rate = k[reactants]^x, where x is the order of the reaction with respect to the given reactant, and k is the rate constant.

· The overall order of a reaction is the sum of all exponents in the rate law.

· The value of the rate constant, k, depends on temperature and activation energy, and its units will vary depending on the reaction order.

· Coefficients of the reactants in the rate limiting step of a mechanism can be used to determine the order of a reaction in the rate law; coefficients from the overall reaction alone CANNOT be used to find the order of a reaction.

CHAPTER 9 FREESTANDING PRACTICE QUESTIONS

1. In the reaction $A + 2B \rightarrow C$, the rate law is experimentally determined to be rate $= k[B]^2$. What happens to the initial rate of reaction when the concentration of A is doubled?

A) The rate doubles.
B) The rate quadruples.
C) The rate is halved.
D) The rate is unchanged.

2. Which of the following statements is always true about the kinetics of a chemical reaction?

A) The rate law includes all reactants in the balanced overall equation.
B) The overall order equals the sum of the reactant coefficients in the overall reaction.
C) The overall order equals the sum of the reactant coefficients in the slow step of the reaction.
D) The structure of the catalyst remains unchanged throughout the reaction progress.

3. Which of the following is represented by a localized minimum in a reaction coordinate diagram?

A) Transition state
B) Product
C) Activated complex
D) Intermediate

4. Which factor always affects both thermodynamic and kinetic properties?

A) Temperature
B) Transition state energy level
C) Reactant coefficients of the overall reaction
D) No single factor always affects both thermodynamics and kinetics.

5. Which of the following best describes the role of pepsin in the process of proteolysis?

A) It stabilizes the structure of the amino acid end products.
B) It lowers the energy requirement needed for the reaction to proceed.
C) It increases the K_{eq} of proteolysis.
D) It lowers the free energy of the peptide reactant.

6. Based on the reaction mechanism shown below, which of the following statements is correct?

$$2\,NO + O_2 \rightarrow 2\,NO_2$$

1) $2\,NO \rightarrow N_2O_2$ (fast)
2) $N_2O_2 + O_2 \rightarrow 2\,NO_2$ (slow)

A) Step 1 is the rate-determining step and the rate of the overall reaction is $k[N_2O_2]$.
B) Step 1 is the rate-determining step and the rate of the overall reaction is $k[NO]^2$.
C) Step 2 is the rate-determining step and the rate of the overall reaction is $k[NO_2]^2$.
D) Step 2 is the rate-determining step and the rate of the overall reaction is $k[N_2O_2][O_2]$.

7. When table sugar is exposed to air it undergoes the following reaction:

$$C_{12}H_{22}O_{11} + 12\,O_2 \rightarrow 12\,CO_2 + 11\,H_2O$$

$$(\Delta G = -5693 \text{ kJ/mol})$$

When this reaction is observed at the macroscopic level, it appears as though nothing is happening, yet one can detect trace amounts of CO_2 and H_2O being formed. These observations are best explained by the fact that the reaction is:

A) thermodynamically favorable but not kinetically favorable.
B) kinetically favorable but not thermodynamically favorable.
C) neither kinetically nor thermodynamically favorable.
D) both kinetically and thermodynamically favorable.

CHAPTER 9 PRACTICE PASSAGE

One way to determine a rate law is to look at the slowest elementary step in a reaction mechanism. The rate law is equal to the rate constant times the initial concentrations of the reactants in the slowest step raised to the power of their coefficients in the balanced equation. If a chemical appears in the rate law raised to the X power, we say the reaction is X order for that chemical.

In cases where the slow step is not the first step, the rate law will likely depend on the concentration of intermediate species. This is experimentally inconvenient, since the concentration of intermediates is not as straightforward to control as starting materials. As such, rate laws are often rewritten substituting terms consisting solely of starting materials, when possible. For example, consider the decomposition of nitramide:

$$O_2NNH_2(aq) \rightarrow N_2O(g) + H_2O(l)$$

Reaction 1

This reaction consists of three elementary steps (shown below), with step 2 as the slow step.

Step 1 (fast equilibrium):
$$O_2NNH_2(aq) \rightleftharpoons O_2NNH^-(aq) + H^+(aq)$$

Step 2 (slow):
$$O_2NNH^-(aq) \rightarrow N_2O(g) + OH^-(aq)$$

Step 3 (fast):
$$H^+(aq) + OH^-(aq) \rightarrow H_2O(l)$$

One could write a valid rate law for this reaction of the form:

$$rate = k[O_2NNH^-]$$

However, the inclusion of the intermediate term is not ideal. The fast equilibrium in Step 1 allows the substitution of $[O_2NNH^-]$ according to the equilibrium condition:

$$K_{eq} = \frac{[O_2NNH^-][H^+]}{[O_2NNH_2]}$$

Solving for $[O_2NNH^-]$, and substituting into the rate law gives an equally valid expression, detailing how the rate may be altered by varying the concentration of starting material and the pH of the reaction mixture:

$$rate = k\left(\frac{K_{eq}[O_2NNH_2]}{[H^+]}\right)$$

The mechanism for this reaction consists of three elementary steps. The first step is an equilibrium reaction with a significant back reaction and the last step is an equilibrium reaction lying so far to the right that we consider it to go to completion:

1. What is the order of the decomposition of nitramide in water with respect to H^+?

   A) Negative first order
   B) One half order
   C) First order
   D) Second order

2. If Step 1 were simply a fast reaction and not a fast equilibrium, what would be the expected rate law for the decomposition of nitramide in water?

   A) Rate $= k[O_2NNH_2]$

   B) Rate $= k[O_2NNH^-]$

   C) Rate $= k[H^+][OH^-]$

   D) Rate $= k\dfrac{[O_2NNH_2]}{[H^+]}$

3. If separately synthesized $Na^+[O_2NNH^-]$ were added to a reaction in progress (assuming total solubility of the salt), what effect would this have on the rate?

   A) No reaction would be observed.
   B) The rate of the reaction would decrease.
   C) The rate of the reaction would increase.
   D) It is impossible to tell without experimental data.

4. If the $[H^+]$ goes up by a factor of four, the reaction rate will

   A) increase by a factor of four.
   B) increase by a factor of two.
   C) decrease by a factor of two.
   D) decrease by a factor of four.

5. Considering Step 1 in isolation, if a known amount of O_2NNH_2 is dissolved in water, which of the following plays a role in determining how fast the reaction reaches equilibrium?

A) The pH of the solution
B) The reaction temperature
C) The magnitude of the equilibrium constant
D) The stability of O_2NNH_2 compared to O_2NNH^- and H^+

6. What is true regarding the enthalpy and entropy changes for Step 3 of the mechanism?

A) $\Delta H > 0, \Delta S > 0$
B) $\Delta H > 0, \Delta S < 0$
C) $\Delta H < 0, \Delta S > 0$
D) $\Delta H < 0, \Delta S < 0$

SOLUTIONS TO CHAPTER 9 FREESTANDING PRACTICE QUESTIONS

1. **D** Since the rate law is independent of [A], (i.e., rate is only dependent on the concentration of B), changing the amount of A will have no effect on the rate.

2. **C** Choice A is incorrect because rate laws are dependent on the slowest step. If a reactant does not participate in the slow step, it will not be included in the overall rate law. Choice B is incorrect because rate laws of overall reactions can only be determined experimentally. Choice D is incorrect because while it is true that a catalyst comes out of a reaction unchanged, it can undergo temporary transformations during the reaction and revert back into its original form at the end. Choice C is the best option because rate laws can be determined from elementary steps of a reaction mechanism by simply raising the reactants to their respective coefficients.

3. **D** It should be noted that choices A and C are the same and should therefore be eliminated. Additionally, transition states are localized maximums, not minimums. Choice B is incorrect because the product for a spontaneous reaction is the absolute minimum and not a localized minimum. Intermediates are formed and then used. They have a certain lifespan represented by a local minimum on the reaction coordinate diagram.

4. **A** Choice B is purely a kinetic factor and can be eliminated. Choice C is eliminated because it dictates the thermodynamic quantity K_{eq} but not necessarily the kinetics of the overall reaction (only of the rate limiting step). Gibbs free energy, a thermodynamic property, is defined as $\Delta G = \Delta H - T\Delta S$, and the Arrhenius equation defines the rate constant k, a kinetic property, as $k = Ae^{(-E_a/RT)}$. Both equations contain the T variable representing temperature. Therefore, choice A is correct and choice D must be incorrect.

5. **B** Pepsin is an enzyme, a biological catalyst. Catalysts lower the activation energy by providing the correct orientation of reactants for a reaction to proceed. Enzymes make a reaction go faster and affect the kinetics of the reaction, making choice B the best answer. Stability of the products, K_{eq}, and free energy of the reactants are all thermodynamic properties, so choices A, C, and D are eliminated.

6. **D** The rate-determining step (RDS) of a reaction mechanism is the slowest step of that mechanism, eliminating choices A and B. The rate law of an elementary step can be determined from the coefficients of the reactants in the elementary step. Because Step 2 is the RDS, the overall rate law will be equivalent to the rate law for the RDS. Therefore, rate $= k[N_2O_2][O_2]$.

7. **A** Given the very negative ΔG value, this is a very thermodynamically favorable, spontaneous chemical reaction (eliminate choice B and C). It is important to make the distinction in this case between kinetics and thermodynamics. The reason only trace amounts of products are formed is that the reaction proceeds at an incredibly slow rate (therefore NOT kinetically favorable) due to a high activation energy.

SOLUTIONS TO CHAPTER 9 PRACTICE PASSAGE

1. **A**   The passage states that if a chemical is raised to the X power, the reaction is X order with respect to that chemical. The rate law can be written as Rate $= k[O_2NNH_2][H^+]^{-1}$, so the reaction is negative first order with respect to H^+.

2. **B**   If the first step was simply a fast step, then we would be able to make the normal assumptions about elementary steps and rate laws. More specifically, the rate law could be determined by the stoichiometry of the slow Step 2, which would yield the rate law in choice B.

3. **C**   Recall that re-writing the rate law in terms of observable starting conditions does not make the rate including $[O_2NNH^-]$ invalid. The two rate laws are equivalent to one another. As such, increasing the concentration of $[O_2NNH^-]$ will increase the reaction rate.

4. **D**   Since $[H^+]$ is in the denominator of the rate law expression and raised to the first power, if $[H^+]$ goes up by a factor of four, the rate will go down by a factor of four.

5. **B**   The question requires an answer related to the kinetics of the reaction. Choices A, C, and D are not kinetic factors. The temperature of a reaction is factored into the rate constant $(k = Ae^{(-E_a/RT)})$, so it will play a role in determining the speed of progress to equilibrium.

6. **D**   Neutralization reactions release large amounts of heat, so ΔH must be less than zero, eliminating choices A and B. From the point of view of entropy, two molecules become one, increasing the order of the system. Moreover, two aqueous species turning into a pure liquid increases order. Therefore, disorder decreases and ΔS must be less than zero.

Chapter 10
Equilibrium

10.1 EQUILIBRIUM

Many reactions are reversible, and situations can occur in which the forward and reverse reactions come into a balance called **equilibrium**. How does equilibrium come about? Before any bonds are broken or made, the reaction flask contains only reactants and no products. As the reaction proceeds, products begin to form and eventually build up, and some of them begin to revert to reactants. That is, once products are formed, both the forward and reverse reactions will occur. Ultimately, the reaction will come to equilibrium, a state at which both the forward and reverse reactions occur at the same constant rate. At equilibrium, the overall concentration of reactants and products remains the same, but at the molecular level, they are continually interconverting. Because the forward and reverse processes balance one another perfectly, we don't observe any net change in concentrations.

> *When a reaction is at equilibrium (and only at equilibrium), the rate of the forward reaction is equal to the rate of the reverse reaction.*

Equilibria occur for *closed systems* (which means no new reactants, products, or other changes are imposed).

The Equilibrium Constant

Each reaction will tend towards its own equilibrium and, for a given temperature, will have an **equilibrium constant**, K_{eq}. For the generic, balanced reaction

$$a \, A + b \, B \; \rightleftharpoons \; c \, C + d \, D$$

the **equilibrium expression** is given by:

$$K_{eq} = \frac{[C]^c [D]^d}{[A]^a [B]^b}$$

This is known as the **mass-action ratio**, where the square brackets represent the molar concentrations at equilibrium.

The constant K is often given a subscript to indicate the type of reaction it represents. For example, K_a (for acids), K_b (for bases), and K_{sp} (for solubility product) are all equilibrium constants. The equilibrium expression is derived from the ratio of the concentration of products to reactants at equilibrium, as follows:

1) Products are in the numerator, and reactants are in the denominator. They are in brackets because the equilibrium expression comes from the *concentrations* (at equilibrium) of the species in the reaction. For two or more reactants or products, multiply the concentrations of each species together.

2) The coefficient of each species in the reaction becomes an exponent on its concentration in the equilibrium expression.

3) Solids and pure liquids are *not* included, because their concentrations don't change. (A substance that's a solid or pure liquid in the reaction is often indicated by an "(s)" or "(l)" subscript, respectively. We're also allowed to omit solvents in dilute solutions because the solvents are in vast excess and their concentrations do not change.)

4) Aqueous dissolved particles are included.

5) If the reaction is gaseous, we can use the partial pressure of each gas as its concentration. The value of the equilibrium constant determined with pressures will be different than with molar concentrations because of their different units. The constant using partial pressures is often termed K_p.

The value of K_{eq} is constant at a given temperature for a particular reaction, no matter what ratio of reactants and products are given at the beginning of the reaction. That is, any closed system will proceed towards its equilibrium ratio of products and reactants even if you start with all products, or a mixture of some reactants and some products. You can even open the flask and add more of any reactant or product, and the system will change until it has reached the K_{eq} ratio. We'll discuss this idea in detail in just a moment, but right now focus on this:

The value of K_{eq} for a given reaction is a constant at a given temperature.

If the temperature changes, then a reaction's K_{eq} value will change.

The value of K_{eq} tells you the direction the reaction favors:

$K_{eq} < 1 \rightarrow$ reaction favors the reactants (i.e., there are more reactants than products at equilibrium)

$K_{eq} = 1 \rightarrow$ reaction has roughly equal amounts of reactants and products

$K_{eq} > 1 \rightarrow$ reaction favors the products (i.e., there are more products than reactants at equilibrium)

Example 10-1: Which of the following expressions gives the equilibrium constant for this reaction:

$$2\,NO \rightleftharpoons N_2 + O_2?$$

A) $[N_2][O_2]/[2\,NO]$
B) $[N_2][O_2]/[NO]^2$
C) $[NO]/[N_2][O_2]$
D) $[NO]^2/[N_2][O_2]$

Solution: The mass-action ratio is products over reactants, so we can immediately eliminate choices C and D. Stoichiometric coefficients become exponents on the concentrations, not coefficients inside the square brackets. Therefore the coefficient of 2 for the reactant NO means the denominator will be $[NO]^2$, so the answer is B.

Example 10-2: A certain reversible reaction comes to equilibrium with high concentration of products and low concentration of reactants. Of the following, which is the most likely value of the equilibrium constant for this reaction?

A) $K_{eq} = -1 \times 10^{-5}$
B) $K_{eq} = 1 \times 10^{-5}$
C) $K_{eq} = 1$
D) $K_{eq} = 1 \times 10^{5}$

Solution: First, eliminate choice A since equilibrium constants are never negative. If the concentration of products is high and the concentration of reactants is low at equilibrium, then the ratio "products over reactants" will have a large value certainly greater than 1. Therefore, choice D is the answer.

Example 10-3: When the reaction $2\,A + B \rightleftharpoons 2\,C$ reaches equilibrium, $[A] = 0.1\ M$ and $[C] = 0.2\ M$. If the value of K_{eq} for this reaction is 8, what is $[B]$ at equilibrium?

A) $0.1\ M$
B) $0.2\ M$
C) $0.4\ M$
D) $0.5\ M$

Solution: The expression for K_{eq} is $\dfrac{[C]^2}{[A]^2[B]}$. We now solve for $[B]$ and substitute in the given values:

$$K_{eq} = \frac{[C]^2}{[A]^2[B]} \rightarrow [B] = \frac{[C]^2}{[A]^2 K_{eq}} = \frac{(0.2)^2}{(0.1)^2(8)} = \frac{2^2}{8} = 0.5$$

The answer is D.

Example 10-4: Which of the following illustrates a chemical system that is at equilibrium?

I. Bubbles forming in solution
II. A solution saturated with solute
III. The ratio of products to reactants remains constant

A) I only
B) II only
C) I and II only
D) II and III only

Solution: *Equilibrium* means that the system no longer changes with time. Both II and III illustrate this; therefore, choice D is best.

Example 10-5: The term *chemical equilibrium* applies to a system:

A) where the forward and reverse reaction have stopped.
B) whose rate law is of zero order.
C) where individual molecules are still reacting, but there is no net change in the system.
D) in which all components are in the same phase.

Solution: A *chemical equilibrium* is a dynamic equilibrium, which means that molecules are still reacting, but there is no net change in the composition of the system. Choice C is the best choice. Choice A describes a static equilibrium, but all chemical equilibria are dynamic. Choice B refers to rate, but all closed reactions may come to equilibrium, regardless of the order of the reaction. Finally, the term describing choice D is *homogeneous*, not *equilibrium*.

10.2 THE REACTION QUOTIENT

The equilibrium constant expression is a ratio: the concentration of the products divided by those of the reactants, each raised to the power equal to its stoichiometric coefficient in the balanced equation. If the reaction is not at equilibrium, the same expression is known simply as the **reaction quotient, Q.** For the generic, balanced reaction

$$a\,A + b\,B \rightleftharpoons c\,C + d\,D$$

the reaction quotient is given by:

$$Q = \frac{[C]^c[D]^d}{[A]^a[B]^b}$$

where the square brackets represent the molar concentrations of the species. The point now is that the concentrations in the expression Q do *not* have to be the concentrations at equilibrium. (If the concentrations are the equilibrium concentrations, the Q will equal K_{eq}.)

Comparing the value of Q to K_{eq} tells us in what direction the reaction will proceed. The reaction will strive to reach a state in which $Q = K_{eq}$. So, if Q is less than K_{eq}, then the reaction will proceed in the forward direction (in order to increase the concentration of the products and decrease the concentration of the reactants) to increase Q to the K_{eq} value. On the other hand, if Q is greater than K_{eq}, then the reaction will proceed in the reverse direction (in order to increase the concentrations of the reactants and decrease the concentrations of the products) to reduce Q to K_{eq}.

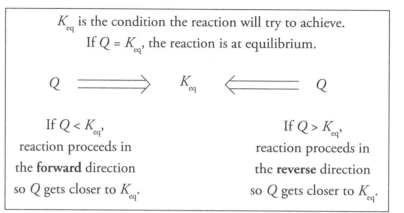

K_{eq} is the condition the reaction will try to achieve.

If $Q = K_{eq}$, the reaction is at equilibrium.

$$Q \implies K_{eq} \impliedby Q$$

If $Q < K_{eq}$,
reaction proceeds in
the **forward** direction
so Q gets closer to K_{eq}.

If $Q > K_{eq}$,
reaction proceeds in
the **reverse** direction
so Q gets closer to K_{eq}.

Example 10-6: The value of the equilibrium constant for the reaction

$$2\ COF_2(g) \rightleftharpoons CO_2(g) + CF_4(g)$$

is $K_{eq} = 2$. If a 1 L reaction container currently holds 1 mole each of CO_2 and CF_4 and 0.5 mole of COF_2, then:

A) the reaction is at equilibrium.
B) the forward reaction will be favored.
C) the reverse reaction will be favored.
D) no prediction can be made without knowing the pressure of the container.

Solution: The expression for Q is $\dfrac{[CO_2][CF_4]}{[COF_2]^2}$. Therefore, the value of Q is:

$$\frac{(1)(1)}{(0.5)^2} = 4$$

Since $Q > K_{eq}$, the reverse reaction will be favored (choice C).

10.3   LE CHÂTELIER'S PRINCIPLE

Le Châtelier's principle states that a system at equilibrium will try to neutralize any imposed change (or stress) in order to reestablish equilibrium. For example, if you add more reactant to a system that is at equilibrium, the system will react by favoring the forward reaction in order to consume that reactant and reestablish equilibrium.

To illustrate, let's look at the Haber process for making ammonia:

$$N_2(g) + 3\ H_2(g) \rightleftharpoons 2\ NH_3(g) + heat$$

Let's assume the reaction is at equilibrium, and see how it reacts to disturbances to the equilibrium by changing the concentration of the species, the pressure, or the temperature.

Adding Ammonia

If we add ammonia, the system is no longer at equilibrium, and there is an excess of product. How can the reaction reestablish equilibrium? By consuming some of the added ammonia, the ratio of products to reactants would decrease towards the equilibrium ratio, so the reverse reaction will be favored (we say the system "shifts to the left"), converting ammonia into nitrogen and hydrogen, until equilibrium is restored.

You can see how this follows from comparing the reaction quotient of the disturbed system to the equilibrium constant. If we add ammonia to the reaction mixture, then $[NH_3]$ increases, and the reaction quotient, Q, becomes greater than K_{eq}. As a result, the reaction will proceed in the reverse direction in order to reduce Q to K_{eq}.

Removing Ammonia

If we remove the product, ammonia, then the forward reaction will be favored—the reaction "shifts to the right"—in order to reach equilibrium again. Again, you can see how this follows from comparing the reaction quotient of the disturbed system to the equilibrium constant. If we remove ammonia from the reaction mixture, then $[NH_3]$ decreases, and the reaction quotient, Q, becomes smaller than K_{eq}. As a result, the reaction will proceed in the forward direction in order to increase Q to K_{eq}.

Adding Hydrogen

If we add some reactant, say $H_2(g)$, then the forward reaction will be favored—the reaction "shifts to the right"—in order to reach equilibrium again. This follows from comparing the reaction quotient of the disturbed system to the equilibrium constant. If we add hydrogen to the reaction mixture, the $[H_2]$ increases, and the reaction quotient, Q, becomes smaller than K_{eq}. As a result, the reaction will proceed in the forward direction in order to increase Q to K_{eq}.

Removing Nitrogen

If we remove some reactant, say $N_2(g)$, then the reverse reaction will be favored—the reaction "shifts to the left"—in order to reach equilibrium again. Again, this follows from comparing the reaction quotient of the disturbed system to the equilibrium constant. If we remove nitrogen from the reaction mixture, then $[N_2]$ decreases, and the reaction quotient, Q, becomes larger than K_{eq}. As a result, the reaction will proceed in the reverse direction in order to decrease Q to K_{eq}.

Changing the Volume of the Reaction Container

The Haber process is a gaseous reaction, so a change in volume will cause the partial pressures of the gases to change. Specifically, a decrease in volume of the reaction container will cause the partial pressures of the gases to increase; an increase in volume reduces the partial pressures of the gases in the mixture. If the number of moles of gas on the left side of the reaction does not equal the number of moles of gas on the right, then a change in pressure due to a change in volume will disrupt the equilibrium ratio, and the system will react to reestablish equilibrium.

How does the system react? Let's first assume the volume is reduced so that the pressure increases. Look back at the equation for the Haber process: There are 4 moles of gas on the reactant side (3 of H_2 plus 1 of N_2) for every 2 moles of NH_3 gas formed. If the reaction shifts to the right, four moles of gas can be condensed into 2 moles, reducing the pressure to reestablish equilibrium. On the other hand, if the volume is increased so that the pressure decreases, the reaction will shift to the left, increasing the pressure to reestablish equilibrium.

To summarize: Consider a gaseous reaction (at equilibrium) with unequal numbers of moles of gas of reactants and products. If the volume is reduced, increasing the pressure, a net reaction occurs favoring the side with the smaller total number of moles of gas. If the volume is expanded, decreasing the pressure, a net reaction occurs favoring the side with the greater total number of moles of gas. (This is only true for reactions involving gases.)

Changing the Temperature of the Reaction Mixture

Heat can be treated as a reactant or a product just like all the chemical reactants and products. Adding or removing heat (by increasing or decreasing the temperature) is like adding or removing any other reagent. Exothermic reactions release heat (which we note on the right side of the equation like a product), and the ΔH will be negative. Endothermic reactions consume heat (which we note on the left side of the equation like a reactant), and the ΔH will be positive.

The Haber process is an exothermic reaction. So, if you increase the temperature at which the reaction takes place once it's reached equilibrium, the reaction will shift to the left in order to consume the extra heat, thereby producing more reactants. If you decrease the temperature at which the reaction takes place once it's reached equilibrium, the reaction will shift to the right in order to produce extra heat, thereby producing more product.

Since the reverse of an exothermic reaction is an endothermic one (and vice versa), every equilibrium reaction involves an exothermic reaction and an endothermic reaction. We can then say this: *Lowering* the temperature favors the *exothermic* reaction, while *raising* the temperature favors the *endothermic* one. Keep in mind that, unlike changes in concentration or pressure, changes in temperature *will* affect the reaction's K_{eq} value, depending on the direction the reaction shifts to reestablish equilibrium.

Note that the above changes are specific to the system *once it is at equilibrium*. The kinetics of the reaction are a different matter. Remember, all reactions proceed faster when the temperature is increased, and this is true for the Haber process. Indeed, in industry this reaction is typically run at around 500°C, despite the fact that the reaction is exothermic. The reason is that a fast reaction with a 10 percent yield of ammonia may end up being better overall than a painfully slow reaction with a 90 percent yield of ammonia. Heating a reaction gets it to equilibrium faster. Once it's there, adding or taking away heat will affect the equilibrium as predicted by Le Châtelier's principle.

Adding an Inert (or Non-Reactive) Gas

What if we injected some helium into a constant volume reaction container? This inert gas doesn't participate in the reaction (and for the MCAT, inert gases don't participate in *any* reaction), so it will change neither the partial pressure nor the concentration of the products or reactants. If neither of these values change, then there is no change in equilibrium.

However, if we inject some helium into a constant pressure container, like one with a movable piston, the extra gas particles will push against the piston, raising it to increase the volume and equilibrate the internal pressure of the gases with external pressure. Since the volume increases, the partial pressures of the gases involved in the reversible reaction will change, thereby causing a shift in the equilibrium as described above for volume changes.

Adding a Catalyst

Adding a catalyst to a reaction that's already at equilibrium has no effect. Because it increases the rate of both the forward and reverse reactions equally, the equilibrium amounts of the species are unchanged. So, the introduction of a catalyst would cause no disturbance. Remember that a catalyst increases the reaction rate but does *not* affect the equilibrium.

Example 10-7: Nitrogen dioxide gas can be formed by the endothermic reaction shown below. Which of the following changes to the equilibrium would *not* increase the formation of NO_2?

$$N_2O_4(g) \rightleftharpoons 2\ NO_2(g) \qquad \Delta H = +58\ kJ$$

A) An increase in the temperature
B) A decrease in the volume of the container
C) Adding additional N_2O_4
D) Removing NO_2 as it is formed

Solution: Since ΔH is positive, this reaction is endothermic, and we can think of heat as a reactant. So if we increase the temperature (thereby "adding a reactant," namely heat), the equilibrium would shift to the right, thus increasing the formation of NO_2. This eliminates choice A. Adding reactant (choice C) or removing product (choice D) would also shift the equilibrium to the right. The answer must be B. A decrease in the volume of the container would increase the pressure of the gases, causing the equilibrium to shift in favor of the side with the fewer number of moles of gases; in this case, that would be to the left.

Example 10-8: If the following endothermic reaction is at equilibrium in a rigid reaction vessel,

$$CH_4(g) + H_2O(g) \rightleftharpoons CO(g) + 3\ H_2(g)$$

which one of the following changes would cause the equilibrium to shift to the right?

A) Adding $Ne(g)$
B) Removing some $H_2O(g)$
C) Increasing the pressure
D) Increasing the temperature

Solution: Choice A would have no effect, since neon is an inert gas and the question states the reaction vessel is rigid, therefore the volume does not change. Removing some reactant (choice B) would shift the equilibrium to the left. An increase in pressure (choice C) would cause the equilibrium to shift in favor of the side with the fewer number of moles of gases; in this case, that would be to the left. The answer must be D. Increasing the temperature of an endothermic reaction will shift the equilibrium toward the products.

Example 10-9: If the reaction

$$2 \, NO(g) + O_2(g) \rightleftharpoons 2 \, NO_2(g) \qquad \Delta H = -120 \text{ kJ}$$

is at equilibrium, which one of the following changes would cause the formation of additional $NO_2(g)$?

A) Increasing the temperature
B) Adding a catalyst
C) Reducing the volume of the reaction container
D) Removing some $NO(g)$

Solution: First, eliminate choice B; adding a catalyst to a reaction that's already at equilibrium has no effect. Now, because ΔH is negative, the reaction is exothermic (that is, we can consider heat to be a product). Increasing the temperature would therefore shift the equilibrium to the left; this eliminates choice A. Also, choice D can be eliminated since removing a reactant shifts the equilibrium to the left. The answer is C: Reducing the volume of the reaction container will increase the pressure, and the equilibrium responds to this stress by favoring the side with the fewer number of moles of gas. In this case, that would mean a shift to the right.

Example 10-10: The Haber process takes place in a container of fixed volume and is at equilibrium:

$$N_2(g) + 3 \, H_2(g) \rightleftharpoons 2 \, NH_3(g) + \text{heat}$$

The amounts of the gases present are measured and recorded. Some additional $N_2(g)$ is then injected into the container, and the system is allowed to return to equilibrium. When it does:

A) the amount of H_2 will be smaller than before, and the amounts of N_2 and NH_3 will be greater than before.
B) the amount of N_2 will be smaller than before, and the amounts of H_2 and NH_3 will be greater than before.
C) the amount of NH_3 will be smaller than before, and the amounts of N_2 and H_2 will be greater than before.
D) the amounts of all three gases will be the same as before.

Solution: The system will respond to this change by shifting to the right to reestablish equilibrium. The added N_2 will mean there's more N_2 in the reaction container, even after equilibrium has been reestablished. Also, the shift toward the product side means there'll be more NH_3 than before as well. And in the shifting of the equilibrium in an attempt to reestablish equilibrium, some of the H_2 got used. As a result, we'd expect that the amount of H_2 will be smaller than before, while the amounts of N_2 and NH_3 are greater than before the injection of the extra N_2 (choice A).

10.4 SOLUTIONS AND SOLUBILITY

Solutions

A **solution** forms when one substance **dissolves** into another, forming a *homogeneous* mixture. The process of dissolving is known as **dissolution**. For example, sugar dissolved into iced tea is a solution (though so is unsweetened tea). A substance present in a relatively smaller proportion is called a **solute**, and a substance present in a relatively greater proportion is called a **solvent**. The process that occurs when the solvent molecules surround the solute molecules is known as **solvation**; if the solvent is water, the process is called **hydration**.

Solutions can involve any of the three phases of matter. For example, you can have a solution of two gases, of a gas in a liquid, of a solid in a liquid, or of a solid in a solid (an **alloy**). However, most of the solutions with which you're familiar have a liquid as the solvent. Salt water has solid salt (NaCl) dissolved into water, seltzer water has carbon dioxide gas dissolved in water, and vinegar has liquid acetic acid dissolved in water. In fact, most of the solutions that you commonly see have water as the solvent: lemonade, tea, soda pop, and corn syrup are examples. When a solution has water as the solvent, it is called an **aqueous** solution.

How do we know which solutes are soluble in which solvents? Well, that's easy:

Like dissolves like.

Solutes will dissolve best in solvents where the intermolecular forces being broken in the solute are being replaced by equal (or stronger) intermolecular forces between the solvent and the solute.

Electrolytes

When ionic substances dissolve, they **dissociate** into ions. Free ions in a solution are called **electrolytes** because the solution can conduct electricity. Some salts dissociate completely into individual ions, while others only partially dissociate (that is, a certain percentage of the ions will remain paired, sticking close to each other rather than being independent and fully surrounded by solvent). Solutes that dissociate completely (like ionic substances) are called **strong electrolytes**, and those that remain ion-paired to some extent are called **weak electrolytes**. (Covalent compounds that don't dissociate into ions are **nonelectrolytes**.) Solutions of strong electrolytes are better conductors of electricity than those of weak electrolytes.

Different ionic compounds will dissociate into different numbers of particles. Some won't dissociate at all, and others will break up into several ions. The **van't Hoff** (or **ionizability**) **factor** (i) tells us how many ions one unit of a substance will produce in a solution. For example,

- $C_6H_{12}O_6$ is non-ionic, so it does not dissociate. Therefore, $i = 1$.
  (Note: The van't Hoff factor for almost all biomolecules—hormones, proteins, steroids—is 1.)
- NaCl dissociates into Na^+ and Cl^-. Therefore, $i = 2$.
- HNO_3 dissociates into H^+ and NO_3^-. Therefore, $i = 2$.
- $CaCl_2$ dissociates into Ca^{2+} and $2 Cl^-$. Therefore, $i = 3$.

Example 10-11: Of the following, which is the *weakest* electrolyte?

10.4

A) NH_4I
B) LiF
C) AgBr
D) H_2O_2

Solution: All ionic compounds, whether soluble or not, are defined as strong electrolytes, so choices A, B, and C are eliminated. Choice D, hydrogen peroxide, is a covalent compound that does not produce an appreciable number of ions upon dissolution and thus is a weak electrolyte. Choice D is the best answer.

The **concentration** of a solution tells you how much solute is dissolved in the solvent (see Section 3.8). A **concentrated** solution has a greater amount of solute per unit volume than a solution that is **dilute**. A **saturated** solution is one in which no more solute will dissolve. At this point, we have reached the **molar solubility** of the solute for that particular solvent, and the reverse process of dissolution, called **precipitation**, occurs at the same rate as dissolving. Both the solid form and the dissolved form of the solute are said to be in **dynamic equilibrium**.

Example 10-12: A researcher adds 0.4 kg of $CaBr_2$ (MW = 200 g/mol) to a large flask and adds enough water to make 10 L of solution.

A) What is the molarity of the calcium bromide in the solution?
B) What is the concentration of bromide ion in the solution?
C) How much water would the researcher need to add to the solution in order to decrease the concentration by a factor of 4?

Solution:

A) Since the molecular weight of $CaBr_2$ is 0.2 kg/mol, a 0.4 kg sample represents 2 moles. Then by definition we have

$$\text{Molarity } (M) = \frac{\#\text{ moles of solute}}{\#\text{ L of solution}} = \frac{2 \text{ mol}}{10 \text{ L}} = 0.2 \ M$$

B) Since $CaBr_2$ dissociates into one Ca^{2+} ion and 2 Br^- ions, the concentration of bromide ion in the solution is 2(0.2 *M*) = 0.4 *M*.

C) Let *x* be the number of liters of additional water added to the solution. If the concentration is to be decreased by a factor of 4 (that is, to 0.05 *M*), then

$$\frac{2 \text{ mol}}{10 \text{ L} + x \text{ L}} = 0.05M \quad \Rightarrow \quad \frac{2}{10 + x} = \frac{5}{100} \quad \Rightarrow \quad x = 30$$

Solubility

Solubility refers to the amount of solute that will saturate a particular solvent. Solubility is specific for the type of solute and solvent. For example, 100 mL of water at 25°C becomes saturated with 40 g of dissolved NaCl, but it would take 150 g of KI to saturate the same volume of water at this temperature. And both of these salts behave differently in methanol than in water. Solubility also varies with temperature, increasing or decreasing with temperature depending upon the solute and solvent as outlined in the first set of solubility rules below.

There are two sets of solubility rules that show up time and time again on the MCAT. The first set governs the general solubility of solids and gases in liquids, as a function of the temperature and pressure. These rules below should be taken as just rules of thumb because they are only 95 percent reliable (still not bad). Memorize the following:

Phase Solubility Rules

1. The solubility of solids in liquids tends to increase with increasing temperature.
2. The solubility of gases in liquids tends to decrease with increasing temperature.
3. The solubility of gases in liquids tends to increase with increasing pressure.

Keep in mind, the solubility of a gas in a liquid is also a function of the partial pressure of that gas above the liquid and the Henry's law constant (Solubility = kP). As partial pressure increases, the quantity of dissolved gas necessarily increases as the equilibrium constant remains unchanged.

The second set governs the solubility of salts in water. Memorize the following too:

Salt Solubility Rules

1. All Group I (Li^+, Na^+, K^+, Rb^+, Cs^+) and ammonium (NH_4^+) salts are *soluble*.

2. All nitrate (NO_3^-), perchlorate (ClO_4^-), and acetate ($C_2H_3O_2^-$) salts are *soluble*.

3. All silver (Ag^+), lead (Pb^{2+}/Pb^{4+}), and mercury (Hg_2^{2+}/Hg^{2+}) salts are *insoluble, except* for their nitrates, perchlorates, and acetates.

Example 10-13: Which of the following salts is expected to be *insoluble* in water?

A) CsOH
B) NH_4NO_3
C) $CaCO_3$
D) $AgClO_4$

Solution: According to the solubility rules for salts in water, choices A, B, and D are expected to be soluble. Choice C is therefore the best answer.

Example 10-14: Which of the following acids could be added to an unknown salt solution and NOT cause precipitation?

A) HCl
B) HI
C) H_2SO_4
D) HNO_3

Solution: According to the solubility rules for salts, all nitrate (NO_3^-) salts are soluble. Therefore, only the addition of nitric acid guarantees that any new ion combination would be soluble. Choice D is the correct answer.

Example 10-15: Which one of the following observations is *inconsistent* with the solubility rules given above?

A) More sugar dissolves in a pot of hot water than in a pot of cold water.
B) Boiler scales are caused by the precipitation of $CaCO_3$ inside plumbing when hot water heaters heat up cold well water.
C) After breathing compressed air at depth, scuba divers that ascend to the surface too quickly risk having air bubbles in their body.
D) Boiling the water before making ice cubes out of it results in clear ice cubes that have no trapped air bubbles.

Solution: Choice A is consistent with phase solubility rule 1, so it is eliminated. Choice C is consistent with phase solubility rule 3, so it is eliminated as well. And finally, choice D is consistent with the second solubility rule 2, so it is also eliminated. Although choice B is a true statement, it is one of those few examples that runs counter to our phase solubility rule 1. Choice B is the correct answer.

Solubility Product Constant

All salts have characteristic solubilities in water. Some, like NaCl, are very soluble, while others, like AgCl, barely dissolve at all. The extent to which a salt will dissolve in water can be determined from its **solubility product constant**, K_{sp}. The solubility product is simply another equilibrium constant, one in which the reactants and products are just the undissolved and dissolved salts.

For example, let's look at the dissolution of magnesium hydroxide in water:

$$Mg(OH)_2(s) \rightleftharpoons Mg^{2+}(aq) + 2\ OH^-(aq)$$

At equilibrium, the solution is *saturated*; the rate at which ions go into solution is equal to the rate at which they precipitate out. The equilibrium expression is

$$K_{sp} = [Mg^{2+}][OH^-]^2$$

Notice that we leave the $Mg(OH)_2$ out of the equilibrium expression because it's a pure solid. (The "concentration of a solid" is meaningless when discussing the equilibrium between a solid and its ions in a saturated aqueous solution.)

Solubility Computations

Let's say you know the K_{sp} for a solid, and you're asked to find out just how much of it can dissolve into water; that is, you're asked to determine the salt's **molar solubility**, the number of moles of that salt that will saturate a liter of water.

To find the solubility of $Mg(OH)_2$, we begin by figuring out how much of each type of ion we'll have once we have x moles of the salt. Since each molecule dissociates into one magnesium ion and two hydroxide ions, if x moles of this salt have dissolved, the solution contains x moles of Mg^{2+} ions and $2x$ moles of OH^- ions:

$$Mg(OH)_2(s) \rightleftharpoons Mg^{2+}(aq) + 2\ OH^-(aq)$$

$$x \rightleftharpoons x + 2x$$

So, if x stands for the number of moles of $Mg(OH)_2$ that have dissolved per liter of saturated solution (which is what we're trying to find), then $[Mg^{2+}] = x$ and $[OH^-] = 2x$. Substituting these into the solubility product expression gives us

$$K_{sp} = [Mg^{2+}][OH^-]^2$$

$$= x(2x)^2 = x(4x^2) = 4x^3$$

It is known that K_{sp} for $Mg(OH)_2$ at 25°C is about 1.6×10^{-11}. So, if we set this equal to $4x^3$, we can solve for x. We get $x \approx 1.6 \times 10^{-4}$. This means that a solution of $Mg(OH)_2$ at 25°C will be saturated at a $Mg(OH)_2$ concentration of $1.6 \times 10^{-4}\ M$.

Example 10-16: The value of the solubility product for copper(I) chloride is $K_{sp} = 1.2 \times 10^{-6}$. Under normal conditions, the maximum concentration of an aqueous CuCl solution will be:

A) less than $10^{-6}\ M$.
B) greater than $10^{-6}\ M$ and less than $10^{-4}\ M$.
C) greater than $10^{-4}\ M$ and less than $10^{-2}\ M$.
D) greater than $10^{-2}\ M$ and less than $10^{-1}\ M$.

Solution: The equilibrium is $CuCl(s) \rightleftharpoons Cu^+(aq) + Cl^-(aq)$. If we let x denote $[Cu^+]$, then we also have $x = [Cl^-]$. Therefore, $K_{sp} = x \times x = x^2$; setting this equal to 1.2×10^{-6}, we find that x is $1.1 \times 10^{-3}\ M$. Therefore, the answer is C.

Example 10-17: The solubility product for lithium phosphate, Li_3PO_4, is $K_{sp} = 2.7 \times 10^{-9}$. How many moles of this salt would be required to form a saturated, 1 L aqueous solution?

Solution: The equilibrium is $Li_3PO_4(s) \rightleftharpoons 3Li^+(aq) + PO_4^{3-}(aq)$. If we let x denote $[PO_4^{3-}]$, then we have $[Li^+] = 3x$. Therefore, $K_{sp} = (3x)^3 \times x = 27x^4$; setting this equal to $2.7 \times 10^{-9} = 27 \times 10^{-10}$ we find that

$$27x^4 = 27 \times 10^{-10} \quad \rightarrow \quad x = (10^{-10})^{1/4} = 10^{-2.5} = 10^{0.5} \times 10^{-3} \approx 3.2 \times 10^{-3}$$

Therefore, 3.2×10^{-3} mol will be required.

10.5 ION PRODUCT

The **ion product** is the reaction quotient for a solubility reaction. That is, while K_{sp} is equal to the product of the concentrations of the ions in solution when the solution is saturated (that is, *at equilibrium*), the ion product—which we'll denote by Q_{sp}—has exactly the same form as the K_{sp} expression, but the concentrations don't have to be those at equilibrium. The reaction quotient allows us to make predictions about what the reaction will do:

$$Q_{sp} < K_{sp} \rightarrow \text{more salt can be dissolved}$$
$$Q_{sp} = K_{sp} \rightarrow \text{solution is saturated}$$
$$Q_{sp} > K_{sp} \rightarrow \text{excess salt will precipitate}$$

For example, let's say we had a liter of solution containing 10^{-4} mol of barium chloride and 10^{-3} mol of sodium sulfate, both of which are soluble salts:

$$BaCl_2(s) \rightarrow Ba^{2+}(aq) + 2\ Cl^-(aq)$$

$$Na_2SO_4(s) \rightarrow 2\ Na^+(aq) + SO_4^{2-}(aq)$$

When you mix two salts in solution, ions can recombine to form new salts, and you have to consider the new salt's K_{sp}. Barium sulfate, $BaSO_4$, is a slightly soluble salt, and at 25°C, its K_{sp} is 1.1×10^{-10}. Its dissolution equilibrium is

$$BaSO_4(s) \rightleftharpoons Ba^{2+}(aq) + SO_4^{2-}(aq)$$

Its ion product is $Q_{sp} = [Ba^{2+}][SO_4^{2-}]$, so in this solution, we have $Q_{sp} = (10^{-4})(10^{-3}) = 10^{-7}$, which is much greater than its K_{sp}. Since $Q_{sp} > K_{sp}$, the reverse reaction would be favored, and $BaSO_4$ would precipitate out of solution.

10.6 THE COMMON-ION EFFECT

Let's consider again a saturated solution of magnesium hydroxide:

$$Mg(OH)_2(s) \rightleftharpoons Mg^{2+}(aq) + 2\ OH^-(aq)$$

What would happen if we now added some sodium hydroxide, NaOH, to this solution? Since NaOH is very soluble in water, it will dissociate completely:

$$NaOH(s) \rightarrow Na^+(aq) + OH^-(aq)$$

The addition of NaOH has caused the amount of hydroxide ion—the **common ion**—in the solution to increase. This disturbs the equilibrium of magnesium hydroxide; since the concentration of a product of that equilibrium is increased, Le Châtelier's principle tells us that the system will react by favoring the reverse reaction, producing solid $Mg(OH)_2$, which will precipitate. Therefore, the molar solubility of the slightly soluble salt [in this case, $Mg(OH)_2$] is decreased by the presence of another solute (in this case, NaOH) that supplies a common ion. This is the **common-ion effect**.

Example 10-18: Barium chromate solid ($K_{sp} = 1.2 \times 10^{-10}$) is at equilibrium with its dissociated ions in an aqueous solution. If calcium chromate ($K_{sp} = 7.1 \times 10^{-4}$) is introduced into the solution, it will cause the molar quantity of:

A) solid barium chromate to increase and barium ion to decrease.
B) solid barium chromate to increase and barium ion to increase.
C) solid barium chromate to decrease and barium ion to decrease.
D) solid barium chromate to decrease and barium ion to increase.

Solution: The answer is A. The introduction of additional chromate ion (CrO_4^{2-})—the common ion—will cause the amount of barium ion in solution to decrease (since the solubility equilibrium of $BaCrO_4$ will be shifted to the left, consuming Ba^{2+}). And, as a result, the amount of solid barium chromate will increase, because some will precipitate.

Example 10-19: A researcher wishes to prepare a saturated solution of a lead compound that contains the greatest concentration of lead(II) ions. Of the following, which should she use?

A) $Pb(OH)_2$ ($K_{sp} = 2.8 \times 10^{-16}$)
B) $PbCl_2$ ($K_{sp} = 1.7 \times 10^{-5}$)
C) PbI_2 ($K_{sp} = 8.7 \times 10^{-9}$)
D) $PbBr_2$ ($K_{sp} = 6.3 \times 10^{-6}$)

Solution: Since the equilibrium had the form $PbX_2(s) \rightleftharpoons Pb^{2+}(aq) + 2\,X^-(aq)$, we have $K_{sp} = [Pb^{2+}][X^-]^2$. Therefore, to maximize $[Pb^{2+}]$, the researcher would want to maximize K_{sp}. Of the choices given, $PbCl_2$ (choice B) has the largest K_{sp} value.

10.7 COMPLEX ION FORMATION AND SOLUBILITY

Complex ions consist of metallic ions surrounded by generally two, four, or six ligands, also known as Lewis bases. Complexed metal ions may have extremely different solubility properties than the "naked," hydrated metal ions. Therefore, the addition of ligands may substantially alter the solubility of simple metal salts. For example, as described by the solubility rules in Section 10.4 above, silver chloride (AgCl) is largely insoluble in water as is evident by its extremely low K_{sp} (1.7×10^{-10}). However, addition of AgCl to an aqueous solution containing ammonia (NH_3) results in greater solubility, owing to the formation of the complex ion $[Ag(NH_3)_2]^+$. The overall effect is described by the equations below:

$$AgCl(s) \rightleftharpoons Ag^+(aq) + Cl^-(aq) \qquad\qquad K_{sp} = 1.6 \times 10^{-10}$$

$$Ag^+(aq) + 2\,NH_3(aq) \rightleftharpoons [Ag(NH_3)_2]^+ (aq) \qquad\qquad K_{eq} = 1.5 \times 10^7$$

Overall: $\quad AgCl(s) + 2\,NH_3(aq) \rightleftharpoons [Ag(NH_3)_2]^+ (aq) + Cl^-(aq) \qquad K_{overall} \approx 10^{-3}$

The inclusion of ammonia in the system greatly increases the propensity of the AgCl(s) to exist as ions in solution. While the final value of K (10^{-3}) is still less than 1, it is several orders of magnitude greater than the initial K_{sp} of AgCl. The dissolution of the initial silver salt can be favored even more by taking advantage of Le Châtelier's Principle through the simple addition of excess ammonia.

10.7

One biological application of complex ion formation is metal-chelation therapy; one of the most commonly used metal chelation agents, ethylenediaminetetraacetic acid (EDTA) is approved by the FDA for the treatment of acute lead poisoning. After the administration of EDTA (generally as a mixed calcium/sodium salt), an equilibrium is established, sequestering the toxic Pb^{2+} ions in the patient's system in a very stable EDTA complex. The following reaction demonstrates the association of fully deprotonated EDTA and Pb^{2+} to form the complex ion:

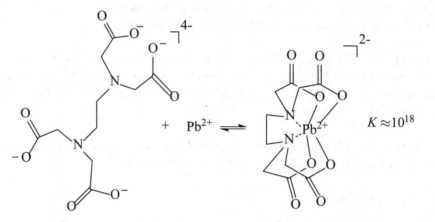

The extremely high equilibrium constant for the formation of the complexed Pb^{2+} ensures that it is prevented from further deleterious interactions with other biological functionalities, and allows its speedy excretion from the body.

10.8 THERMODYNAMICS AND EQUILIBRIUM

In Section 6.5 on Gibbs Free Energy, we saw that if ΔG was negative we could expect a reaction to proceed spontaneously in the forward direction, with the opposite being true for the case in which ΔG is positive. When a system proceeds in one direction or another there is necessarily a change in the relative values of products and reactants that redefine ΔG, and the reaction proceeds until ΔG is equal to 0 and equilibrium is achieved. Therefore, there must be a relationship between ΔG and the reaction quotient Q, as well as the equilibrium constant K_{eq}. This relationship is given in the following equation.

$$\Delta G = \Delta G^\circ + RT \ln Q$$

As the superscript denotes, ΔG° is the Gibbs free energy for a reaction under standard conditions. You may recall from Section 10.2 that when $Q = K$ the reaction is at equilibrium. Since ΔG is always equal to zero at equilibrium we can change the equation to

$$0 = \Delta G^\circ + RT \ln K_{eq}$$

or

$$\Delta G^\circ = -RT \ln K_{eq}$$

10.8

It is important to draw the distinction between ΔG and $\Delta G°$. Whereas ΔG is a statement of spontaneity of a reaction in one direction or another, $\Delta G°$ is, as seen in its relation to K_{eq}, a statement of the relative proportions of products and reactants present at equilibrium. The standard state $\Delta G°$ for a reaction only describes a reaction at one specific temperature, pressure, and set of concentrations, whereas ΔG changes with changing reaction composition until it reaches zero. From the above relationship, we can surmise the following:

$\Delta G° < 0$; $K_{eq} > 1$, products are favored at equilibrium

$\Delta G° = 0$; $K_{eq} = 1$, products and reactants are present in roughly equal amounts at equilibrium

$\Delta G° > 0$; $K_{eq} < 1$, reactants are favored at equilibrium

The difference between the heights of the reactants and products on any reaction coordinate diagram is $\Delta G°$. As we know from analyzing these plots if the reactants are higher than the products, we expect the products to be favored. This would give us the expected negative value of $\Delta G°$, and likewise a value of K_{eq} greater than 1.

10.8

Chapter 10 Summary

- The equilibrium constant dictates the relative ratios of products to reactant when a system is at equilibrium.

- For $a\text{A} + b\text{B} \rightarrow c\text{C} + d\text{D}$: $K_{eq} = [\text{C}]^c[\text{D}]^d / [\text{A}]^a[\text{B}]^b$

- Pure solids and liquids are not included in the equilbrium expression.

- If $K > 1$, products are favored. If $K < 1$ reactants are favored.

- The reaction quotient, Q, is a ratio of products and reactants with the same form as K, but can be used when the reaction isn't at equilibrium. If $Q < K$, the reaction will proceed in the forward reaction; if $Q > K$, the reaction will proceed in the reverse direction until equilibrium is achieved.

- The only factor that changes the equilibrium constant is temperature.

- Changing the concentrations of the products or reactants of a reaction at equilibrium will force the system to shift according to Le Châtelier's principle.

- Increasing the temperature of a system at equilibrium favors the products in an endothermic reaction and the reactants in an exothermic reaction. Decreasing the temperature will have the opposite effect on both types of reactions.

- In a gaseous reaction, increasing the pressure by decreasing the volume favors the side of the reaction with fewer moles of gas. Decreasing the pressure has the opposite effect.

- An electrolyte is a solute that produces free ions in solution. Strong electrolytes produce more ions in solution than weak electrolytes.

- The van't Hoff (or ionizability) factor, i, tells us how many ions one unit of a substance will produce in solution.

- All Group I, ammonium, nitrate, perchlorate, and acetate salts are completely soluble. All silver, lead, and mercury salts are insoluble, except when they are paired with nitrate, perchlorate, or acetate.

- The solubility of solids in liquids increases with increasing temperature.

- The solubility of gases in liquids decreases with increasing temperature and increases with increasing pressure.

- The amount of a salt that can be dissolved in a solute is given by its solubility product constant (K_{sp}).

- For a reaction at equilibrium under standard conditions, $\Delta G° = -RT\ln K_{eq}$.

- For a reaction under non-standard conditions, ΔG can be calculated using $\Delta G = \Delta G° + RT\ln Q$.

CHAPTER 10 FREESTANDING PRACTICE QUESTIONS

1. Which of the following manipulations is capable of changing the K_{eq} of the reaction shown below?

$$N_2(g) + 3 H_2(g) \rightleftharpoons 2 NH_3(g)$$

   A) Doubling the concentrations of $N_2(g)$, $H_2(g)$, and $NH_3(g)$
   B) Tripling the volume of the reaction container
   C) Increasing the pressure from 1 to 2 atm
   D) Decreasing the temperature to from 298 K to 273 K

2. A group of scientists is studying the dynamics of the acetic acid dissociation below and bring the process to equilibrium under standard conditions. If the scientists then add 35 g of sodium acetate to the reaction container, which of the following will be true?

$$CH_3COOH(aq) \rightleftharpoons CH_3COO^-(aq) + H^+(aq)$$

   A) $Q > K_{eq}$ and the reaction will move in reverse.
   B) $Q < K_{eq}$ and the reaction will move forward.
   C) $Q > K_{eq}$ and the reaction will move forward.
   D) $Q < K_{eq}$ and the reaction will move in reverse.

3. Given the following equilibrium:

$$N_2(g) + 3 H_2(g) \rightleftharpoons 2 NH_3(g) \quad \Delta H = -91.8 kJ$$

   How would an increase in temperature affect the concentration of N_2 at equilibrium?

   A) The concentration of N_2 will increase because of an increase in K_{eq}.
   B) The concentration of N_2 will decrease because of an increase in K_{eq}.
   C) The concentration of N_2 will increase because of a decrease in K_{eq}.
   D) The concentration of N_2 will remain unchanged.

4. Na_2SO_4 is soluble in water. If $NaCl(s)$ is added to a solution of $Na_2SO_4(aq)$ so that the concentration of Na^+ doubles, then the:

   A) solubility constant of Na_2SO_4 increases while that of NaCl decreases.
   B) solubility constants of Na_2SO_4 and NaCl both decrease.
   C) solubility of Na_2SO_4 and NaCl both decrease.
   D) solubility of Na_2SO_4 decreases while that of NaCl increases.

5. The equilibrium expression below corresponds to which of the following reactions?

$$K_{eq} = \frac{(P_{SO_2})^2 \cdot P_{O_2}}{(P_{SO_3})^2}$$

   A) $2 SO_2(aq) + O_2(g) \rightleftharpoons 2 SO_3(aq)$
   B) $2 SO_3(aq) \rightleftharpoons 2 SO_2(aq) + O_2(g)$
   C) $2 SO_2(g) + O_2(g) \rightleftharpoons 2 SO_3(g)$
   D) $2 SO_3(g) \rightleftharpoons 2 SO_2(g) + O_2(g)$

6. Which of the following salts is least soluble in water?

   A) PbI_2 ($K_{sp} = 7.9 \times 10^{-9}$)
   B) $Mg(OH)_2$ ($K_{sp} = 6.3 \times 10^{-10}$)
   C) $Zn(IO_3)_2$ ($K_{sp} = 3.9 \times 10^{-6}$)
   D) SrF_2 ($K_{sp} = 2.6 \times 10^{-9}$)

7. The water solubility of $MgSO_4$ is approximately 25 g/100 mL at 20°C. Compared to a 0.25 g/mL solution of $MgSO_4$ prepared at 20°C, a 0.25 g/mL solution prepared at 37°C will:

   A) dissolve faster and have the same concentration of ions in solution.
   B) dissolve faster and have a higher concentration of ions in solution.
   C) dissolve slower and have a lower concentration of ions in solution.
   D) dissolve slower and have the same concentration of ions in solution.

8. If the K_{sp} of KI is 1.45×10^{-6} in propanol at 25°C, what would the K_{sp} of KI be in propane at the same temperature?

A) 1.84
B) 2.90×10^{-3}
C) 1.81×10^{-6}
D) 7.56×10^{-23}

9. The K_{sp} of NaCl in water is 35.9 at 25°C. If 500 mL of 12 M NaOH(aq) and 500 mL of 12 M HCl(aq) solution both at 25°C are combined, what would best describe the resulting solution?

A) A small amount of NaCl(s) would precipitate.
B) There will be a 6 M aqueous solution of NaCl.
C) Enthalpy and entropy would increase.
D) The resulting solution would be slightly basic.

CHAPTER 10 PRACTICE PASSAGE

A chemist attempted to measure and contrast the solubilities of carbon dioxide, hydrogen sulfide, and nitrogen in water, noting that carbon dioxide and hydrogen sulfide undergo dissociation reactions in solution:

$$CO_2(g) \rightleftharpoons CO_2(aq)$$

$$CO_2(aq) + H_2O(l) \rightleftharpoons H_2CO_3(aq)$$

$$H_2CO_3(aq) \rightleftharpoons H^+(aq) + HCO_3^-(aq)$$

$$HCO_3^-(aq) \rightleftharpoons H^+(aq) + CO_3^{2-}(aq)$$

$$H_2S(g) \rightleftharpoons H_2S(aq)$$

$$H_2S(aq) \rightleftharpoons H^+(aq) + HS^-(aq)$$

She constructed a special 10.0 L airtight vessel equipped with a very sensitive closed-end manometer.

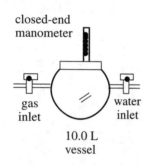

During each trial of the experiment, she evacuated all of the air from the system and then filled the vessel with one of the gases above to a pressure of 760 torr at 25°C. Five liters of water were then slowly pumped into the vessel without allowing any of the gas to escape. After the system was allowed to reach equilibrium for one hour, the pressure of the gas over the water was recorded. Each gas was analyzed three times in this manner.

Trial Set	Gas	Measured pressure (in torr)
1	CO$_2$	1312
2		1307
3		1311
1	H$_2$S	1357
2		1363
3		1363
1	N$_2$	1520
2		1519
3		1521

Note that the vapor pressure of pure water is 24 torr at 25°C.

1. Which of the following statements is NOT a valid rationalization for the results of the solubility tests?

A) CO$_2$ and H$_2$S are polar molecules, while N$_2$ is not.
B) CO$_2$ and H$_2$S produce ions in solution, while N$_2$ does not.
C) CO$_2$ and H$_2$S are weak acids in water, N$_2$ is not.
D) The covalent bonds in CO$_2$ and H$_2$S are polar, but those in N$_2$ are not.

2. Approximately how many moles of gas were used in each trial of the set #3 experiments?

A) 0.1
B) 0.4
C) 0.8
D) 1.0

3. The addition of sodium hydroxide to the water used in these experiments would:

A) increase the solubility of CO$_2$.
B) decrease the solubility of CO$_2$.
C) increase the K for the dissolution of CO$_2$.
D) decrease the K for the dissolution of CO$_2$.

4. If an equivalent experiment using the chemically inert gas SF_6 were carried out, resulting in a final reading of 1224 torr, what might be calculated as the approximate molar solubility of SF_6 in water at 25°C? (R = ~62 torr·L/mol·K)

A) 1.7×10^{-4} mol/L
B) 1.7×10^{-3} mol/L
C) 1.7×10^{-2} mol/L
D) 1.7×10^{-1} mol/L

5. Which one of the following conclusions is NOT supported by the data in this experiment?

A) At 25°C, CO_2 is more soluble than H_2S or N_2.
B) Nitrogen gas is completely insoluble in water.
C) The pH values of the CO_2 and H_2S solutions are less than 8.
D) Molecules without overall dipole moments may be significantly soluble in water.

6. A fourth set of experiments was performed using molecular oxygen. If the value of the K_{diss} for oxygen in water was determined to be 0.02 at 25°C, then the value of K_{diss} of O_2 could be 0.01 in a solution with:

A) lower pressure.
B) higher temperature.
C) an $O_2(g)$ to $O_2(aq)$ catalyst.
D) more water.

SOLUTIONS TO CHAPTER 10 FREESTANDING PRACTICE QUESTIONS

1. **D**   Equilibrium constants are specific to a single temperature and standard state free energy change according to: $\Delta G° = -RT\ln K$. Altering temperature is the only answer choice that can change the reaction's K_{eq}.

2. **A** K_{eq} = [products]/[reactants] when both reactant and product concentrations are those at equilibrium. Q = [products]/[reactants] regardless of whether reactant and product concentrations are those at equilibrium. The addition of sodium acetate essentially translates into the addition of acetate ion, a product in this equilibrium. As a result of such an addition, $Q > K_{eq}$ and products are present in excess of equilibrium values. Le Châtelier's principle states that net reverse movement is created when the concentration of products is increased in an equilibrium system.

3. **C**   Since the reaction is exothermic, an increase in temperature will shift the equilibrium to the left, and the concentration of N_2 will increase, eliminating choices B and D. For exothermic reactions, an increase in temperature will decrease the K_{eq}, eliminating choice A and making choice C the correct answer.

4. **C**   Solubility constants, like all equilibrium constants, are functions of temperature only. This eliminates choices A and B. Given the equilibria:

    $$Na_2SO_4(s) \rightleftharpoons 2\,Na^+\,(aq) + SO_4^{2-}\,(aq)$$
    $$NaCl(s) \rightleftharpoons Na^+\,(aq) + Cl^-\,(aq)$$

    Na^+ is a common ion to both systems. Increasing Na^+ concentration will decrease the solubility of both salts, eliminating choice D and making choice C the best answer.

5. **D**   The expression is in terms of partial pressure, so all components must be gaseous, eliminating choices A and B. An equilibrium expression has products in the numerator and reactants in the denominator, eliminating choice C. The exponents correspond to the stoichiometric coefficients of the balanced equation, so choice D is correct.

6. **B**   All of the compounds are composed of one cation and two anions, so comparing K_{sp} values will give relative solubility. Since the question asks for an extreme, the middle values of the variable cannot be correct, eliminating choices A and D. The compound with the lowest K_{sp} value will have the lowest solubility because for all the compounds, K_{sp} = [cation][anion]^2. Therefore, choice B is correct.

7. **A**   This is a two-by-two problem. First, consider rate. Any time temperature is increased, the reaction kinetics increase. In this case, the salt will dissolve faster, eliminating choices C and D. An increase in temperature generally causes an increase in the solubility of solids in liquids. However, both solutions contain the same amount of $MgSO_4$ that does not exceed the maximum solubility at either temperature. Therefore, the concentrations of ions will be the same, eliminating choice B.

8. **D** The golden rule of solubility is "like dissolves like." Potassium iodide is a salt held together by ionic forces and therefore comprised of charged ions. A salt will dissolve in a polar solvent better than a non-polar solvent. Propanol has a polar –OH group whereas propane is completely non-polar. Therefore, KI must have a smaller K_{sp} in propane than in propanol. The only answer that has a smaller K_{sp} value is choice D.

9. **B** Neutralizations are exothermic and form salt and water. The starting 500 mL solutions contain 6 moles each of NaOH and HCl. The final solution will be 1 L of 6 M NaCl(aq):

$$6 \ HCl(aq) + 6 \ NaOH(aq) \rightarrow 6 \ NaCl(aq) + 6 \ H_2O(l)$$

Although the reaction quotient of NaCl in this resulting solution will slightly exceed K_{sp}:

$$Q = [Na^+][Cl^-] = [6][6] = 36$$

the temperature will be significantly increased, allowing more NaCl to dissolve (K_{sp} will increase with temperature), eliminating choice A. Choice C is eliminated because enthalpy significantly decreases as heat is given off in this exothermic reaction. Choice D is eliminated because NaCl is a neutral salt.

SOLUTIONS TO CHAPTER 10 PRACTICE PASSAGE

1. **A** The solubility tests indicate CO_2 and H_2S are more soluble in water than N_2. The passage tells us that CO_2 and H_2S dissolve in water to produce hydrogen ions (choices B and C are OK). The covalent bonds in CO_2 and H_2S are all highly polar (choice D is OK), but CO_2 is a linear, symmetric molecule. So while each C–O bond is polar, overall the CO_2 molecule is nonpolar.

2. **B** Initially, the flasks were filled with 10.0 L of gas at 25°C and 760 torr. For the sake of simplicity, we can assume that we are dealing with gases at STP (0°C and 760 torr) because the difference in the volume of a gas at STP and at 25°C and 760 torr (as in this experiment) is less than 10%. Since 1.0 mole of any ideal gas occupies a volume of 22.4 L at STP, 10.0 L of a gas is a little less than half a mole, or about 0.4 mol.

3. **A** The equilibrium and solubility constants of any substance are only functions of temperature, not pressure, concentration, or the presence of a catalyst (choices C and D are eliminated). Based upon the equilibrium reactions given in the passage, the addition of hydroxide would consume H^+. As $[H^+]$ decreases, the equilibrium of reaction (2) and (3) shifts to the right. This in turn, decreases the concentration of carbonic acid, H_2CO_3, which causes reaction (1) to shift to the right, driving more $CO_2(g)$ to dissolve in the solution.

4. **C**   When the 10 L flask is charged with SF_6, the number of moles can be calculated from the ideal gas law as follows:

$$\frac{(760 \text{ torr})(10 \text{ L})}{(62 \text{ torr·L/mol·K})(298 \text{ K})} = n$$

62×298 can be rounded to $62 \times 300 = (60 \times 300) + (2 \times 300) = 18600$.

$$\frac{7600}{18600} = \frac{76}{186} = \frac{38}{93} = \sim 0.4 \text{ mol}$$

The number of moles left undissolved can be calculated, using 1200 torr as the partial pressure of SF_6 after the subtraction of the 24 torr allotted to the partial pressure of water:

$$\frac{(1200 \text{ torr})(5 \text{ L})}{(62 \text{ torr·L/mol·K})(298 \text{ K})} = n$$

$$\frac{1200}{\sim 12 \times 300} = \sim \frac{100}{300} = 0.33 \text{ mol}$$

From these numbers ~0.07 mol of SF_6 is soluble in 5 L of water, giving a value of ~0.014 mol/L, and making choice C the best answer.

5. **B**   Choices A, C, and D are all statements that are substantiated by the passage. If the initial pressure of 10.0 L of nitrogen was 760 torr, then decreasing the volume of insoluble gas to 5.00 L, the pressure should be 1520 torr. However, we cannot neglect the contribution of the vapor pressure of water, which is 24 torr at 25°C. Therefore, if N_2 were completely insoluble in water, the observed pressure should be 1520 torr + 24 torr = 1544 torr. A pressure less than this (as in this experiment) indicates that some nitrogen has dissolved into the solution.

6. **B**   This question is just trying to see if you recall that the equilibrium constant for any reaction will only change with a change in temperature (choice B). Other factors, like pressure and reactant concentration shift the equilibrium so that the original value of K is re-established.

Chapter 11
Acids and Bases

11.1 DEFINITIONS

There are two important definitions of acids and bases you should be familiar with for the MCAT.

Brønsted-Lowry Acids and Bases

Brønsted and Lowry offered the following definitions:

Acids are proton (H⁺) donors.
Bases are proton (H⁺) acceptors.

→ protons

While the often seen hydroxide ions qualify as Brønsted-Lowry bases, many other compounds fit this definition as well. Since a Brønsted-Lowry base is any substance that is capable of accepting a proton, any anion or any neutral species with a lone pair of electrons can function as a base.

If we consider the reversible reaction below:

$$H_2CO_3 + H_2O \rightleftharpoons H_3O^+ + HCO_3^-$$

then according to the Brønsted-Lowry definition, H_2CO_3 and H_3O^+ are acids and HCO_3^- and H_2O are bases. The Brønsted-Lowry definitions of acid and bases is the most important one for MCAT General Chemistry.

→ e⁻ pairs

Lewis Acids and Bases

Lewis's definitions of acids and bases are broader:

Lewis acids are electron-pair acceptors.
Lewis bases are electron-pair donors.

If we consider the reversible reaction below:

$$AlCl_3 + H_2O \rightleftharpoons (AlCl_3OH)^- + H^+$$

then according to the Lewis definition, $AlCl_3$ and H^+ are acids because they accept electron pairs; H_2O and $(AlCl_3OH)^-$ are bases because they donate electron pairs. Lewis acid/base reactions frequently result in the formation of coordinate covalent bonds, as discussed in Chapter 5. For example, in the reaction above, water acts as a Lewis base since it donates both of the electrons involved in the coordinate covalent bond between OH^- and $AlCl_3$. $AlCl_3$ acts as a Lewis acid, since it accepts the electrons involved in this bond.

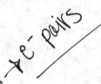

11.2 CONJUGATE ACIDS AND BASES

When a Brønsted-Lowry acid donates an H^+, the remaining structure is called the conjugate base of the acid. Likewise, when a Brønsted-Lowry base bonds with an H^+ in solution, this new species is called the conjugate acid of the base. To illustrate these definitions, consider this reaction:

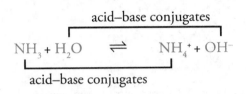

Considering only the forward direction, NH_3 is the base and H_2O is the acid. The products are the conjugate acid and conjugate base of the reactants: NH_4^+ is the conjugate acid of NH_3, and OH^- is the conjugate base of H_2O:

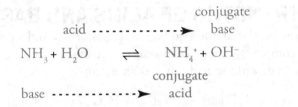

Now consider the reverse reaction in which NH_4^+ is the acid and OH^- is the base. The conjugates are the same as for the forward reaction: NH_3 is the conjugate base of NH_4^+, and H_2O is the conjugate acid of OH^-:

$$\text{conjugate base} \xleftarrow{\quad\quad} \text{acid}$$
$$NH_3 + H_2O \rightleftharpoons NH_4^+ + OH^-$$
$$\text{conjugate acid} \xleftarrow{\quad\quad} \text{base}$$

The difference between a Brønsted-Lowry acid and its conjugate base is that the base is missing an H^+. The difference between a Brønsted-Lowry base and its conjugate acid is that the acid has an extra H^+.

forming conjugates:

$$\text{acid} \underset{+\,H^+}{\overset{-\,H^+}{\rightleftharpoons}} \text{base}$$

Example 11-1: Which one of the following can behave as a Brønsted-Lowry acid but not a Lewis acid?

A) CF_4
B) $NaAlCl_4$
C)   HF
D) Br_2

Solution: A Brønsted-Lowry acid donates an H⁺, while a Lewis acid accepts a pair of electrons. Since a Brønsted-Lowry acid must have an H in the first place, only choice C can be the answer.

Example 11-2: What is the conjugate base of HBrO (hypobromous acid)?

- A) H^+
- B) H_2BrO_2
- C) H_2BrO^+
- D) BrO^-

Solution: To form the conjugate base of an acid, simply remove an H⁺. Therefore, the conjugate base of HBrO is BrO^-, choice D.

11.3 THE STRENGTHS OF ACIDS AND BASES

Brønsted-Lowry acids can be placed into two big categories: *strong* and *weak*. Whether an acid is strong or weak depends on how completely it ionizes in water. A **strong** acid is one that dissociates completely (or very nearly so) in water; hydrochloric acid, HCl, is an example:

$$HCl(aq) + H_2O(l) \rightarrow H_3O^+(aq) + Cl^-(aq)$$

This reaction goes essentially to completion.

On the other hand, hydrofluoric acid, HF, is an example of a **weak** acid, since its dissociation in water,

$$HF(aq) + H_2O(l) \rightleftharpoons H_3O^+(aq) + F^-(aq)$$

does not go to completion; most of the HF remains undissociated.

If we use HA to denote a generic acid, its dissociation in water has the form

$$HA(aq) + H_2O(l) \rightleftharpoons H_3O^+(aq) + A^-(aq)$$

The strength of the acid is directly related to how much the products are favored over the reactants. The equilibrium expression for this reaction is

$$K_a = \frac{[H_3O^+][A^-]}{[HA]}$$

This is written as K_a, rather than K_{eq}, to emphasize that this is the equilibrium expression for an acid-dissociation reaction. In fact, K_a is known as the **acid-ionization** (or **acid-dissociation**) **constant** of the acid (HA). If $K_a > 1$, then the products are favored, and we say the acid is strong; if $K_a < 1$ then the reactants are favored and the acid is weak. We can also rank the relative strengths of acids by comparing their K_a values: The larger the K_a value, the stronger the acid; the smaller the K_a value, the weaker the acid.

The acids for which $K_a > 1$—the strong acids—are so few that you should memorize them:

Common Strong Acids	
Hydroiodic acid	HI
Hydrobromic acid	HBr
Hydrochloric acid	HCl
Perchloric acid	$HClO_4$
Sulfuric acid	H_2SO_4
Nitric acid	HNO_3

The values of K_a for these acids are so large that most tables of acid ionization constants don't even list them. On the MCAT, you may assume that any acid that's not in this list is a weak acid. (Other acids that fit the definition of *strong* are so uncommon that it's very unlikely they'd appear on the test. For example, $HClO_3$ has a K_a of 10, and could be considered strong, but it is definitely one of the weaker strong acids and is not likely to appear on the MCAT.)

Example 11-3: In a 1 M aqueous solution of boric acid (H_3BO_3, $K_a = 5.8 \times 10^{-10}$), which of the following species will be present in solution in the greatest quantity?

A) H_3BO_3
B) $H_2BO_3^-$
C) HBO_3^{2-}
D) H_3O^+

Solution: The equilibrium here is $H_3BO_3(aq) + H_2O(l) \rightleftharpoons H_3O^+(aq) + H_2BO_3^-(aq)$. Boric acid is a weak acid (it's not on the list of strong acids), so the equilibrium lies to the left (also, notice how small its K_a value is). So, there'll be very few H_3O^+ or $H_2BO_3^-$ ions in solution but plenty of undissociated H_3BO_3. The answer is A.

Example 11-4: Of the following, which statement best explains why HF is a weak acid, but HCl, HBr, and HI are strong acids?

A)   F has a greater ionization energy than Cl, Br, or I.
B)   F has a larger radius than Cl, Br, or I.
C) F^- has a larger radius than Cl^-, Br^-, I^-.
D) F^- has a smaller radius than Cl^-, Br^-, I^-.

Solution: F is smaller than Cl, Br, or I (eliminating choices B and C). Ionization energy is associated with forming a cation from a neutral atom, and has no bearing here. Choice D is therefore correct. The more stable an acid's conjugate base is, the stronger the acid. Larger anions are better able to spread out their negative charge, making them more stable. HF is the weakest of the H-X acids because it has the least stable conjugate base due to its size.

Example 11-5: Of the following acids, which one would dissociate to the greatest extent (in water)?

A) HCN (hydrocyanic acid), $K_a = 6.2 \times 10^{-10}$
B) HNCO (cyanic acid), $K_a = 3.3 \times 10^{-4}$
C) HClO (hypochlorous acid), $K_a = 2.9 \times 10^{-8}$
D) HBrO (hypobromous acid), $K_a = 2.2 \times 10^{-9}$

Solution: The acid that would dissociate to the greatest extent would have the greatest K_a value. Of the choices given, HNCO (choice B) has the greatest K_a value.

We can apply the same ideas as above to identify strong and weak *bases*. If we use B to denote a generic base, its dissolution in water has the form

$$B(aq) + H_2O(l) \rightleftharpoons HB^+(aq) + OH^-(aq)$$

The strength of the base is directly related to how much the products are favored over the reactants. If we write the equilibrium constant for this reaction, we get:

$$K_b = \frac{[HB^+][OH^-]}{[B]}$$

This is written as K_b, rather than K_{eq}, to emphasize that this is the equilibrium expression for a base-dissociation reaction. In fact, K_b is known as the **base-ionization** (or **base-dissociation**) **constant**. We can rank the relative strengths of bases by comparing their K_b values: The larger the K_b value, the stronger the base; the smaller the K_b value, the weaker the base.

For the MCAT and general chemistry, you should know about the following strong bases that may be used in aqueous solutions:

Common Strong Bases
Group 1 hydroxides (For example, NaOH)
Group 1 oxides (For example, Li_2O)
Some group 2 hydroxides ($Ba(OH)_2$, $Sr(OH)_2$, $Ca(OH)_2$)
Metal amides (For example, $NaNH_2$)

Weak bases include ammonia (NH_3) and amines, as well as the conjugate bases of many weak acids, as we'll discuss below.

The Relative Strengths of Conjugate Acid–Base Pairs

Let's once again look at the dissociation of HCl in water:

$$HCl(aq) + H_2O(l) \rightarrow H_3O^+(aq) + Cl^-(aq)$$

no basic properties

The chloride ion (Cl^-) is the conjugate base of HCl. Since this reaction goes to completion, there must be no reverse reaction. Therefore, Cl^- has no tendency to accept a proton and thus does not act as a base. The conjugate base of a strong acid has no basic properties in water.

On the other hand, hydrofluoric acid, HF, is a weak acid since its dissociation is not complete:

$$HF(aq) + H_2O(l) \rightleftharpoons H_3O^+(aq) + F^-(aq)$$

Since the reverse reaction does take place to a significant extent, the conjugate base of HF, the fluoride ion, F^-, *does* have some tendency to accept a proton, and so behaves as a weak base. The conjugate base of a weak acid is a weak base.

In fact, the weaker the acid, the more the reverse reaction is favored, and the stronger its conjugate base. For example, hydrocyanic acid (HCN) has a K_a value of about 5×10^{-10}, which is much smaller than that of hydrofluoric acid ($K_a \approx 7 \times 10^{-4}$). Therefore, the conjugate base of HCN, the cyanide ion, CN^-, is a stronger base than F^-.

The same ideas can be applied to bases:

1) The conjugate acid of a strong base has no acidic properties in water. For example, the conjugate acid of LiOH is Li^+, which does not act as an acid in water.
2) The conjugate acid of a weak base is a weak acid (and the weaker the base, the stronger the conjugate acid). For example, the conjugate acid of NH_3 is NH_4^+, which is a weak acid.

Example 11-6: Of the following anions, which is the strongest base?

A) I^-
B) CN^-
C) NO_3^-
D) Br^-

Solution: Here's another way to ask the same question: Which of the following anions has the weakest conjugate acid? Since HI, HNO_3, and HBr are all strong acids, while HCN is a weak acid, CN^- (choice B) has the weakest conjugate acid, and is thus the strongest base.

Example 11-7: Of the following, which acid has the weakest conjugate base?

A) $HClO_4$
B) HCOOH
C) H_3PO_4
D) H_2CO_3

Solution: Here's another way to ask the same question: Which of the following acids is the strongest? Thought about this way, the answer's easy. Perchloric acid, choice A, is the only strong acid in the list.

Amphoteric Substances

Take a look at the dissociation of carbonic acid (H_2CO_3), a weak acid:

$$H_2CO_3(aq) + H_2O(l) \rightleftharpoons H_3O^+(aq) + HCO_3^-(aq) \quad (K_a = 4.5 \times 10^{-7})$$

The conjugate base of carbonic acid is HCO_3^-, which also has an ionizable proton. Carbonic acid is said to be **polyprotic**, because it has more than one proton to donate.

Let's look at how the conjugate base of carbonic acid dissociates:

$$HCO_3^-(aq) + H_2O(l) \rightleftharpoons H_3O^+(aq) + CO_3^{2-}(aq) \quad (K_a = 4.8 \times 10^{-11})$$

In the first reaction, HCO_3^- acts as a base, but in the second reaction it acts as an acid. Whenever a substance can act as either an acid or a base, we say that it is **amphoteric**. The conjugate base of a weak polyprotic acid is always amphoteric, because it can either donate or accept another proton. Also notice that HCO_3^- is a weaker acid than H_2CO_3; in general, every time a polyprotic acid donates a proton, the resulting species will be a weaker acid than its predecessor.

11.4   THE ION-PRODUCT CONSTANT OF WATER

Water is amphoteric. It reacts with itself in a Brønsted-Lowry acid-base reaction, one molecule acting as the acid, the other as the base:

$$H_2O(l) + H_2O(l) \rightleftharpoons H_3O^+(aq) + OH^-(aq)$$

This is called the autoionization (or self-ionization) of water. The equilibrium expression is

$$K_w = [H_3O^+][OH^-]$$

This is written as K_w, rather than K_{eq}, to emphasize that this is the equilibrium expression for the autoionization of water; K_w is known as the ion-product constant of water. Only a very small fraction of the water molecules will undergo this reaction, and it's known that at 25°C,

$$K_w = 1.0 \times 10^{-14}$$

(Like all other equilibrium constants, K_w varies with temperature; it increases as the temperature increases. However, because 25°C is so common, this is the value you should memorize.) Since the number of H_3O^+ ions in pure water will be equal to the number of OH^- ions, if we call each of their concentrations x, then $x^2 = K_w$, which gives $x = 1 \times 10^{-7}$. That is, the concentration of both types of ions in pure water is 1×10^{-7} M. (In addition, K_w is constant at a given temperature, regardless of the H_3O^+ concentration.)

If the introduction of an acid increases the concentration of H_3O^+ ions, then the equilibrium is disturbed, and the reverse reaction is favored, decreasing the concentration of OH^- ions. Similarly, if the introduction of a base increases the concentration of OH^- ions, then the equilibrium is again disturbed; the reverse reaction is favored, decreasing the concentration of H_3O^+ ions. However, in either case, the product of $[H_3O^+]$ and $[OH^-]$ will remain equal to K_w.

For example, suppose we add 0.002 moles of HCl to water to create a 1-liter solution. Since the dissociation of HCl goes to completion (it's a strong acid), it will create 0.002 moles of H_3O^+ ions, so $[H_3O^+] = 0.002$ M. Since H_3O^+ concentration has been increased, we expect the OH^- concentration to decrease, which it does:

$$[OH^-] = \frac{K_w}{[H_3O^+]} = \frac{1 \times 10^{-14}}{2 \times 10^{-3}} = 5 \times 10^{-12}\, M$$

11.5 pH

The pH scale measures the concentration of H^+ (or H_3O^+) ions in a solution. Because the molarity of H^+ tends to be quite small and can vary over many orders of magnitude, the pH scale is logarithmic:

$$pH = -\log[H^+]$$

This formula implies that $[H^+] = 10^{-pH}$. Since $[H^+] = 10^{-7}$ M in pure water, the pH of water is 7. At 25°C, this defines a pH neutral solution. If $[H^+]$ is greater than 10^{-7} M, then the pH will be less than 7, and the solution is said to be acidic. If $[H^+]$ is less than 10^{-7} M, the pH will be greater than 7, and the solution is basic (or alkaline). Notice that a *low* pH means a *high* $[H^+]$ and the solution is *acidic*; a *high* pH means a *low* $[H^+]$ and the solution is basic.

$$pH > 7 \qquad \text{basic solution}$$
$$pH = 7 \qquad \text{neutral solution}$$
$$pH < 7 \qquad \text{acidic solution}$$

The range of the pH scale for most solutions falls between 0 and 14, but some strong acids and bases extend the scale past this range. For example, a 10 M solution of HCl will fully dissociate into H^+ and Cl^-. Therefore, the $[H^+] = 10$ M, and the pH = –1.

An alternate measurement expresses the acidity or basicity in terms of the hydroxide ion concentration, $[OH^-]$, by using pOH. The same formula applies for hydroxide ions as for hydrogen ions.

$$pOH = -\log[OH^-]$$

This formula implies that $[OH^-] = 10^{-pOH}$.

Acids and bases are inversely related: the greater the concentration of H^+ ions, the lower the concentration of OH^- ions, and vice versa. Since $[H^+][OH^-] = 10^{-14}$ at 25°C, the values of pH and pOH satisfy a special relationship at 25°C:

$$pH + pOH = 14$$

So, if you know the pOH of a solution, you can find the pH, and vice versa. For example, if the pH of a solution is 5, then the pOH must be 9. If the pOH of a solution is 2, then the pH must be 12.

On the MCAT, it will be helpful to be able to figure out the pH even in cases where the H^+ concentration isn't exactly equal to the whole-number power of 10. In general, if y is a number between 1 and 10, and you're told that $[H^+] = y \times 10^{-n}$ (where n is a whole number) then the pH will be between $(n-1)$ and n. For example, if $[H^+] = 6.2 \times 10^{-5}$, then the pH is between 4 and 5.

Relationships Between Conjugates

pK_a and pK_b

The definitions of pH and pOH both involve a negative logarithm. In general, "p" of something is equal to the $-\log$ of that something. Therefore, the following definitions won't be surprising:

$$pK_a = -\log K_a$$

$$pK_b = -\log K_b$$

Because H^+ concentrations are generally very small and can vary over such a wide range, the pH scale gives us more convenient numbers to work with. The same is true for pK_a and pK_b. Remember that the larger the K_a value, the stronger the acid. Since "p" means "take the negative log of…," the *lower* the pK_a value, the stronger the acid. For example, acetic acid (CH_3COOH) has a K_a of 1.75×10^{-5}, and hypochlorous acid (HClO) has a K_a of 2.9×10^{-8}. Since the K_a of acetic acid is larger than that of hypochlorous acid, we know this means that more molecules of acetic acid than hypochlorous acid will dissociate into ions in aqueous solution. In other words, acetic acid is stronger than hypochlorous acid. The pK_a of acetic acid is 4.8, and the pK_a of hypochlorous acid is 7.5. The acid with the lower pK_a value is the stronger acid. The same logic applies to pK_b: the lower the pK_b value, the stronger the base.

K_a and K_b

Let's now look at the relationship between the K_a and the K_b for an acid-base conjugate pair by working through an example question. Let K_a be the acid-dissociation constant for formic acid (HCOOH) and let K_b stand for the base-dissociation constant of its conjugate base (the formate ion, $HCOO^-$). If K_a is equal to 5.6×10^{-11}, what is $K_a \times K_b$?

The equilibrium for the dissociation of HCOOH is

$$HCOOH(aq) + H_2O(l) \rightleftharpoons H_3O^+(aq) + HCOO^-(aq)$$

so

$$K_a = \frac{[H_3O^+][HCOO^-]}{[HCOOH]}$$

The equilibrium for the dissociation of $HCOO^-$ is

$$HCOO^-(aq) + H_2O(l) \rightleftharpoons HCOOH(aq) + OH^-(aq)$$

so

$$K_b = \frac{[HCOOH][OH^-]}{[HCOO^-]}$$

Therefore,

$$K_aK_b = \frac{[H_3O^+][HCOO^-]}{[HCOOH]} \times \frac{[HCOOH][OH^-]}{[HCOO^-]} = [H_3O^+][OH^-]$$

We now immediately recognize this product as K_w, the ion-product constant of water, whose value (at 25°C) is 1×10^{-14}.

This calculation wasn't special for HCOOH; we can see that the same thing will happen for any acid and its conjugate base. So, for any acid-base conjugate pair, we'll have

$$K_aK_b = K_w = 1 \times 10^{-14}$$

This gives us a way to quantitatively relate the strength of an acid and its conjugate base. For example, the value of K_a for HF is about 7×10^{-4}; therefore, the value of K_b for its conjugate base, F^-, is about 1.4×10^{-11}. For HCN, $K_a \approx 5 \times 10^{-10}$, so K_b for CN^- is 2×10^{-5}.

It also follows from our definitions and logarithm algebra that for an acid-base conjugate pair at 25°C, we'll have

$$pK_a + pK_b = 14$$

Example 11-8: Of the following liquids, which one contains the lowest concentration of H_3O^+ ions?

A) Lemon juice (pH = 2.3)
B) Blood (pH = 7.4)
C) Seawater (pH = 8.5)
D) Coffee (pH = 5.1)

Solution: Since $pH = -\log[H_3O^+]$, we know that $[H_3O^+] = 1/10^{pH}$. This fraction is smallest when the pH is greatest. Of the choices given, seawater (choice C) has the highest pH.

Example 11-9: What is the pH of a solution at 25°C whose hydroxide ion concentration is 1×10^{-4} M?

Solution: Since pOH = $-\log[OH^-]$, we know that pOH = 4. Therefore, the pH is 10.

Example 11-10: Orange juice has a pH of 3.5. What is its $[H^+]$?

Solution: Because pH = $-\log[H^+]$, we know that $[H^+] = 10^{-pH}$. For orange juice, then, we have $[H^+] = 10^{-3.5} = 10^{0.5-4} = 10^{0.5} \times 10^{-4} = \sqrt{10} \times 10^{-4} \approx 3.2 \times 10^{-4}$ M.

Example 11-11: If 99% of the H_3O^+ ions are removed from a solution whose pH was originally 3, what will be its new pH?

Solution: If 99% of the H_3O^+ ions are removed, then only 1% remain. This means that the number of H_3O^+ ions is now only 1/100 of the original. If $[H_3O^+]$ is decreased by a factor of 100, then the pH is *increased* by 2—to pH 5 in this case—since log 100 = 2.

Example 11-12: Given that the self-ionization of water is endothermic, what is the value of the sum pH + pOH at 50°C?

$$H_2O(l) + H_2O(l) \rightleftharpoons H_3O^+(aq) + OH^-(aq)$$

A) Less than 14
B) Equal to 14
C) Greater than 14
D) Cannot determine from the information given

Solution: This is a Le Châtelier's principle question in disguise. Imagine we start at equilibrium at 25°C; which way would the self-ionization reaction shift if we increase the temperature to 50°C? Since the question tells us this reaction is endothermic, we can consider heat as one of the reactants, and therefore an increase in temperature would cause the system to shift to the right. Shifting to the right means that at equilibrium, $[H^+]$ and $[OH^-]$ will increase. So pH and pOH will both be *lower* than 7 at 50°C, and the sum of pH and pOH will be less than 14 at 50°C. Choice A is the correct answer.

pH Calculations

For Strong Acids

Strong acids dissociate completely, so the hydrogen ion concentration will be the same as the concentration of the acid. That means that you can calculate the pH directly from the molarity of the solution. For example, a 0.01 M solution of HCl will have $[H^+] = 0.01$ M and pH = 2.

For Weak Acids

Weak acids come to equilibrium with their dissociated ions. In fact, for a weak acid at equilibrium, the concentration of undissociated acid will be much greater than the concentration of hydrogen ion. To get the pH of a weak acid solution, you need to use the equilibrium expression.

Let's say you add 0.2 mol of HCN (hydrocyanic acid, a weak acid) to water to create a 1-liter solution, and you want to find the pH. Initially, [HCN] = 0.2 M, and none of it has dissociated. If x moles of HCN are dissociated at equilibrium, then the equilibrium concentration of HCN is 0.2 − x. Now, since each molecule of HCN dissociates into one H^+ ion and one CN^- ion, if x moles of HCN have dissociated, there'll be x moles of H^+ and x moles of CN^-:

	HCN	$\rightleftharpoons$	H^+	+	CN^-
initial:	0.2 M		0 M		0 M
at equilibrium:	(0.2 − x) M		x M		x M

(Actually, the initial concentration of H^+ is 10^{-7} M, but it's so small that it can be neglected for this calculation.) Our goal is to find x, because once we know [H^+], we'll know the pH. So, we set up the equilibrium expression:

$$K_a = \frac{[H^+][CN^-]}{[HCN]} = \frac{x^2}{0.2 - x}$$

It's known that the value of K_a for HCN is 4.9×10^{-10}. Because the K_a is so small, not that much of the HCN is going to dissociate. (This assumption, that x added to or subtracted from a number is negligible, is always a good one when $K < 10^{-4}$ [the usual case found on the MCAT].) That is, we can assume that x is going to be a very small number, insignificant compared to 0.2; therefore, the value (0.2 − x) is almost exactly the same as 0.2. By substituting 0.2 for (0.2 − x), we can solve the equation above for x:

$$\frac{x^2}{0.2} \approx 4.9 \times 10^{-10}$$
$$x^2 \approx 1 \times 10^{-10}$$
$$\therefore x \approx 1 \times 10^{-5}$$

Since [H^+] is approximately 1×10^{-5} M, the pH is about 5.

We simplified the computation by assuming that the concentration of hydrogen ion [H^+] was insignificant compared to the concentration of undissociated acid [HCN]. Since it turned out that [H^+] $\approx 10^{-5}$ M, which is much less than [HCN] = 0.2 M, our assumption was valid. On the MCAT, you should always simplify the math wherever possible.

Example 11-13: If 0.7 mol of benzoic acid (C_6H_5COOH, $K_a = 6.6 \times 10^{-5}$) is added to water to create a 1-liter solution, what will be the pH?

Solution: Initially $[C_6H_5COOH] = 0.7\ M$, and none of it has dissociated. If x moles of C_6H_5COOH are dissociated at equilibrium, then the equilibrium concentration of C_6H_5COOH is $0.7 - x$. Now, since each molecule of C_6H_5COOH dissociates into one H^+ ion and one $C_6H_5COO^-$ ion, if x moles of C_6H_5COOH have dissociated, there'll be x moles of H^+ and x moles of $C_6H_5COO^-$:

	C_6H_5COOH	$\rightleftharpoons$	H^+	+	$C_6H_5COO^-$
initial:	$0.7\ M$		$0\ M$		$0\ M$
at equilibrium:	$(0.7 - x)\ M$		$x\ M$		$x\ M$

(Again, the initial concentration of H^+ is $10^{-7}\ M$, but it's so small that it can be neglected.) Our goal is to find x, because once we know $[H^+]$, we'll know the pH. So, we set up the equilibrium expression:

$$K_a = \frac{[H^+][C_6H_5COO^-]}{[C_6H_5COOH]} = \frac{x^2}{0.7 - x} \approx \frac{x^2}{0.7}$$

and then solve the equation for x:

$$\frac{x^2}{0.7} \approx 6.6 \times 10^{-5}$$
$$x^2 \approx 4.6 \times 10^{-5} = 46 \times 10^{-6}$$
$$\therefore x \approx 7 \times 10^{-3}$$

Since $[H^+]$ is approximately $7 \times 10^{-3}\ M \approx 10^{-2}\ M$, the pH is a little more than 2, say 2.2.

11.6 NEUTRALIZATION REACTIONS

When an acid and a base are combined, they will react in what is called a **neutralization reaction**. Oftentimes this reaction will produce a salt and water. Here's an example:

$$HCl\ +\ NaOH\ \rightarrow\ NaCl\ +\ H_2O$$

$$\text{acid} \qquad \text{base} \qquad \text{salt} \qquad \text{water}$$

This type of reaction takes place when, for example, you take an antacid to relieve excess stomach acid. The antacid is a weak base, usually carbonate, that reacts in the stomach to neutralize acid.

If equimolar amounts of a strong acid and strong base react (as in the example above), the resulting solution will be pH neutral. However, if the reaction involves a weak acid or weak base, the resulting solution will not be pH neutral.

No matter how weak an acid or base is, when mixed with an equimolar amount of a strong base or acid, we can expect complete neutralization. It has been found experimentally that all neutralizations have the same exothermic "heat of neutralization," the energy released from the reaction that is the same for all neutralizations: $H^+ + OH^- \rightarrow H_2O$.

As you can see from the reaction above, equal molar amounts of HCl and NaOH are needed to complete the neutralization. To determine just how much base (B) to add to an acidic solution (or how much acid (A) to add to a basic solution) in order to cause complete neutralization, we just use the following formula:

$$a \times [A] \times V_A = b \times [B] \times V_B$$

where a is the number of acidic hydrogens per formula unit and b is a constant that tells us how many H^+ ions the base can accept.

For example, let's calculate how much 0.1 M NaOH solution is needed to neutralize 40 mL of a 0.3 M HCl solution:

$$V_B = \frac{a \times [A] \times V_A}{b \times [B]} = \frac{1 \times (0.3\,M) \times (40\text{ mL})}{1 \times (0.1\,M)} = 120\text{ mL}$$

Example 11-14: Binary mixtures of equal moles of which of the following acid-base combinations will lead to a complete (99+%) neutralization reaction?

   I.   HCl and NaOH
  II.   HF and NH_3
 III. HNO_3 and $NaHCO_3$

  A)   I only
  B)   I and II only
  C)   II and III only
  D)   I, II, and III

Solution: Remember, regardless of the strengths of the acids and bases, all neutralization reactions go to completion. Choice D is the correct answer.

11.6

11.7 HYDROLYSIS OF SALTS

A **salt** is an ionic compound, consisting of a cation and an anion. In water, the salt dissociates into ions, and depending on how these ions react with water, the resulting solution will be either acidic, basic, or pH neutral. To make the prediction, we notice that there are essentially two possibilities for both the cation and the anion in a salt:

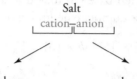

Salt
cation—anion

doesn't react with water
(for example: Group 1 cations,
larger Group 2 cations)

or

stronger acid than water
(for example: NH_4^+, Be^{2+},
Cu^{2+}, Zn^{2+}, Al^{3+}, Cr^{3+}, Fe^{3+})

doesn't react with water
(for example: conjugate base
of a strong acid)

or

stronger base than water
(for example: conjugate base
of a weak acid)

Whether the salt solution will be acidic, basic, or pH neutral depends on which combination of possibilities (four total) from the diagram above applies. The reaction of a substance—such as a salt or an ion—with water is called a hydrolysis reaction, a more general use of the term since the water molecule may not be split. Let's look at some examples.

If we dissolve NaCl in water, Na^+ and Cl^- ions go into solution. Na^+ ions are Group 1 ions and do not react with water. Since Cl^- is the conjugate base of a strong acid (HCl), it also doesn't react with water. These ions just become hydrated (surrounded by water molecules). Therefore, the solution will be pH neutral.

How about NH_4Cl? In solution it will break into NH_4^+ and Cl^-. The ammonium ion is a stronger acid than water (it's the conjugate acid of NH_3, a weak base), and Cl^- will not react with water. As a result, a solution of this salt will be acidic (note the formation of hydronium ions as products), and have a pH less than 7. NH_4Cl is called an acidic salt.

$$NH_4^+(aq) + H_2O(l) \rightleftharpoons NH_3(aq) + H_3O^+(aq)$$

Now let's consider sodium acetate, $Na(CH_3COO)$. In solution it will break into Na^+ and CH_3COO^-. Na^+ is a Group 1 cation and does not react with water. However, CH_3COO^- is a stronger base than water since it's the conjugate base of acetic acid (CH_3COOH), a weak acid. Therefore, a solution of the salt will be basic (note the formation of hydroxide ions as products), and have a pH greater than 7. $NaCH_3COO$ is a basic salt.

$$CH_3COO^-(aq) + H_2O(l) \rightleftharpoons CH_3COOH(aq) + OH^-(aq)$$

11.7

Finally, let's consider NH_4CN. In solution it will break into NH_4^+ and CN^-. NH_4^+ is a stronger acid than water, and CN^- is a stronger base than water (it's the conjugate base of HCN, a weak acid). So, which one wins? In a case like this, we need to know the K_a value for the reaction of the cation with water with the K_b value for the reaction of the anion with water and compare these values. Since

$$NH_4^+(aq) + H_2O(l) \rightleftharpoons NH_3(aq) + H_3O^+(aq) \quad (K_a = 6.3 \times 10^{-10})$$

$$CN^-(aq) + H_2O(l) \rightleftharpoons HCN(aq) + OH^-(aq) \quad (K_b = 1.6 \times 10^{-5})$$

we see that in this case K_b of CN^- > K_a of NH_4^+, so the forward reaction of the second reaction will dominate the forward reaction of the first reaction, and the solution will be basic. It is highly unlikely that the level of analysis required for this final example will be required on the MCAT, but you *should* be able to *qualitatively* predict the pH of any salt solution the MCAT throws at you.

Example 11-15: Which of the following salts will produce a basic solution when added to pure water?

A) KCl
B) NaClO
C) NH_4Cl
D) $MgBr_2$

Solution: NaClO (choice B) will dissociate into Na^+ and ClO^-. Na^+ is a Group 1 cation, so it has no effect on the pH. However, ClO^-, the hypochlorite ion, is the conjugate base of a weak acid, HClO (hypochlorous acid). Therefore, the solution will be basic. The salt in choices A will have no effect on the pH, and the salts in choice C and D will leave the solution acidic (since NH_4^+ is the conjugate acid of a weak base, NH_3, and Mg^{2+} will react with water to form the weak base $Mg(OH)_2$).

Example 11-16: Which of the following is an acidic salt?

A) KNO_3
B) $SrCl_2$
C) $CuCl_2$
D) $Ba(CH_3COO)_2$

Solution: Cu^{2+} is a stronger acid than water, so $CuCl_2$ (choice C) is an acidic salt. The salts in choices A and B are neither acidic nor basic, and choice D is a basic salt.

11.7

11.8 BUFFER SOLUTIONS

A **buffer** is a solution that resists changing pH when a small amount of acid or base is added. The buffering capacity comes from the presence of a weak acid and its conjugate base (or a weak base and its conjugate acid) in roughly equal concentrations.

One type of buffer is made from a weak acid and a salt of its conjugate base. To illustrate how a buffer works, let's look at a specific example and add 0.1 mol of acetic acid (CH_3COOH) and 0.1 mol of sodium acetate ($NaCH_3COO$) to water to obtain a 1-liter solution. Since acetic acid is a weak acid ($K_a = 1.75 \times 10^{-5}$), it will partially dissociate to give some acetate (CH_3COO^-) ions. However, the salt is soluble and will dissociate completely to give plenty of acetate ions. The addition of this common ion will shift the acid dissociation to the left, so the equilibrium concentrations of undissociated acetic acid molecules and acetate ions will be essentially equal to their initial concentrations, 0.1 M.

$$CH_3COOH + H_2O \rightleftharpoons H_3O^+ + CH_3COO^-$$

Since buffer solutions are designed to resist changes in pH, let's first figure out the pH of this solution. Writing the expression for the equilibrium constant gives

$$K_a = \frac{[H_3O^+][CH_3COO^-]}{[CH_3COOH]}$$

which we can solve for $[H_3O^+]$:

$$[H_3O^+] = \frac{K_a[CH_3COOH]}{[CH_3COO^-]} \qquad \text{(Equation 1)}$$

Since the equilibrium concentrations of both CH_3COOH and CH_3COO^- are 0.1 M, this equation tells us that

$$[H_3O^+] = \frac{K_a[CH_3COOH]}{[CH_3COO^-]} = \frac{K_a(0.1\,M)}{0.1\,M} = 1.75 \times 10^{-5}$$

and pH $= -\log[H_3O^+]$, so

$$pH = -\log(1.75 \times 10^{-5})$$
$$pH = 4.76$$

Okay, now let's see what happens if we add a little bit of strong acid—HCl, for example. If we add, say, 0.005 mol of HCl, it will dissociate completely in solution into 0.005 mol of H^+ ions and 0.005 mol of Cl^- ions. The Cl^- ions will have no effect on the equilibrium, but the added H^+ (or H_3O^+) ions will. Adding a product shifts the equilibrium to the left, and the acetate ions react with the additional H_3O^+ ions to produce additional acetic acid molecules. As a result, the concentration of acetate ions will drop by 0.005, from 0.1 M to 0.095 M; the concentration of acetic acid will increase by 0.005, from 0.1 M to 0.105 M. Let's now use Equation (1) above to find the new pH:

$$[H_3O^+] = \frac{K_a[CH_3COOH]}{[CH_3COO^-]} = \frac{K_a(0.105\,M)}{0.095\,M} = 1.75 \times 10^{-5}(1.105) = 1.93 \times 10^{-5}$$

and

$$pH = -\log(1.93 \times 10^{-5})$$
$$pH = 4.71$$

Notice that the pH dropped from 4.76 to 4.71, a decrease of just 0.05. If we had added this HCl to a liter of pure water, the pH would have dropped from 7 to 2.3, a *much* larger decrease! The buffer solution we created was effective at resisting a large drop in pH because it had enough base (in the form of acetate ions in this case) to neutralize the added acid.

Now let's see what happens if we add a little bit of strong base—KOH, for example. If we add, say, 0.005 mol of KOH, it will dissociate completely in solution into 0.005 mol of K^+ ions and 0.005 mol of OH^- ions. The K^+ ions will have no effect, but the added OH^- ions will shift the equilibrium to the right, since they'll react with acetic acid molecules to produce more acetate ions ($CH_3COOH + OH^- \rightarrow CH_3COO^- + H_2O$). As a result, the concentration of acetic acid will drop by 0.005, from 0.1 M to 0.095 M; the concentration of acetate ions will increase by 0.005, from 0.1 M to 0.105 M. Let's again use Equation (1) above to find the new pH:

$$[H_3O^+] = \frac{K_a[CH_3COOH]}{[CH_3COO^-]} = \frac{K_a(0.095\ M)}{0.105\ M} = 1.75 \times 10^{-5}(0.905) = 1.58 \times 10^{-5}$$

and

$$pH = -\log(1.58 \times 10^{-5})$$
$$pH = 4.80$$

Notice that the pH increased from 4.76 to 4.80, an increase of just 0.04. If we had added this KOH to a liter of pure water, the pH would have increased from 7 to 11.7, a much larger increase! The buffer solution we created was effective at resisting a large rise in pH because it had enough acid to neutralize the added base.

If we generalize Equation (1) to any buffer solution containing a weak acid and a salt of its conjugate base, we get $[H_3O^+] = K_a([\text{weak acid}]/[\text{conjugate base}])$. Taking the –log of both sides give us the

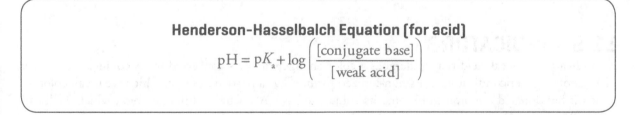

Henderson-Hasselbalch Equation (for acid)

$$pH = pK_a + \log\left(\frac{[\text{conjugate base}]}{[\text{weak acid}]}\right)$$

To design a buffer solution, we choose a weak acid whose pK_a is as close to the desired pH as possible. An ideal buffer would have [weak acid] = [conjugate base], so pH = pK_a. If no weak acid has the exact pK_a needed, just adjust the initial concentrations of the weak acid and conjugate base accordingly.

We can also design a buffer solution by choosing a weak base (and a salt of its conjugate acid) such that the pK_b value of the base is as close to the desired pOH as possible. The version of the Henderson-Hasselbalch equation in this situation looks like this:

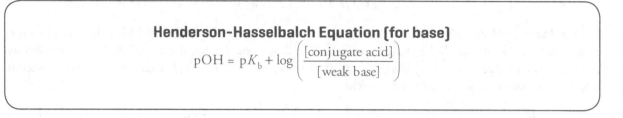

Henderson-Hasselbalch Equation (for base)

$$pOH = pK_b + \log\left(\frac{[\text{conjugate acid}]}{[\text{weak base}]}\right)$$

Example 11-17: Which of the following compounds could be added to a solution of HCN to create a buffer?

A) HNO_3
B) $CaCl_2$
C) NaCN
D) KOH

Solution: HCN is a weak acid, so we'd look for a salt of its conjugate base, CN^-. Choice C, NaCN, is such a salt.

Example 11-18: As hydrogen ions are added to an acidic buffer solution, what happens to the concentrations of undissociated acid and conjugate base?

Solution: The conjugate base, A^-, reacts with the added H^+ to form HA, so the conjugate base decreases and the undissociated acid increases.

Example 11-19: As hydrogen ions are added to an alkaline buffer solution, what happens to the concentrations of base and conjugate acid?

Solution: The base, B, reacts with the added H^+ to form HB^+, so the base decreases and the conjugate acid increases.

11.9 INDICATORS

An **indicator** is a weak acid that undergoes a color change when it's converted to its conjugate base. Let HA denote a generic indicator. In its non-ionized form, it has a particular color, which we'll call color #1. When it has donated a proton to become its conjugate base, A^-, it has a different color, which we'll call color #2.

Indicator

$$HA + H_2O \rightleftharpoons H_3O^+ + A^-$$

color #1   color #2

Under what conditions would an indicator change its color? What if an indicator were added to an acidic solution—that is, one whose pH were quite low due to a high concentration of H_3O^+ ions? Then according to Le Châtelier, the indicator's equilibrium would shift to the left, and the indicator would display color #1. Conversely, if the indicator were added to a basic solution (that is, one with plenty of OH^- ions), the amount of H_3O^+ would decrease, and the indicator's equilibrium would be shifted to the right, causing it to display color #2. We can make this discussion a little more precise.

Take the expression for the indicator's equilibrium constant, $K_a = [H_3O^+][A^-]/[HA]$ and easily rearrange it into

$$\frac{[H_3O^+]}{K_a} = \frac{[HA]}{[A^-]}$$

Written this way, we can see that

- If $[H_3O^+] \gg K_a$, then $[HA] \gg [A^-]$, so we'd see color #1.
- If $[H_3O^+] \approx K_a$, then $[HA] \approx [A^-]$, so we'd see a mix of colors #1 & #2.
- If $[H_3O^+] \ll K_a$, then $[HA] \ll [A^-]$, so we'd see color #2.

Note that the indicator changes color within a fairly short pH range, about 2 units:

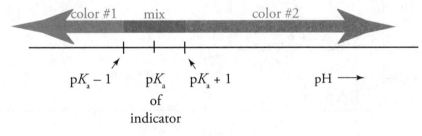

Therefore, if we want our indicator to be useful, we need to select one whose pK_a value is convenient for our purposes. For example, phenolphthalein is an indicator with a pK_a value of about 9.0. When added to a solution whose pH is less than 8, it remains colorless. However, if the solution's pH is above 10, it will turn a deep magenta. (For 8 < pH < 10, the solution will be a paler pink.) Thus, phenolphthalein can be used to differentiate between a solution whose pH is, say, 7 from one whose pH is 11. However, the indicator methyl orange could not distinguish between two such solutions: It would be yellow at pH 7 and yellow at pH 11. Methyl orange has a pK_a of about 3.8, so it changes color around pH 4.

Note: The $pK_a \pm 1$ range for an indicator's color change is convenient and typical, but it's not a hard-and-fast rule. Some indicators (like methyl orange) have a color-change range of only 1.2 (rather than 2) pH units. Also, some indicators have more than just two colors. Polyprotic indicators, like thymol blue and bromocesol green, can change color more than once, and can therefore exhibit more than two distinct colors.

11.10   ACID-BASE TITRATIONS

An **acid-base titration** is an experimental technique used to determine the identity of an unknown weak acid (or weak base) by determining its pK_a (or pK_b). Titrations can also be used to determine the concentration of *any* acid or base solution (whether it be known or unknown). The procedure consists of adding a strong acid (or a strong base) of *known* identity and concentration—the **titrant**—to a solution containing the unknown base (or acid). (One never titrates an acid with an acid or a base with a base.) While the titrant is added in small, discrete amounts, the pH of the solution is recorded (with a pH meter).

If we plot the data points (the pH value vs. the volume of titrant added), we obtain a graph called a titration curve. Let's consider a specific example: the titration of HF (a weak acid) with NaOH (a strong base).

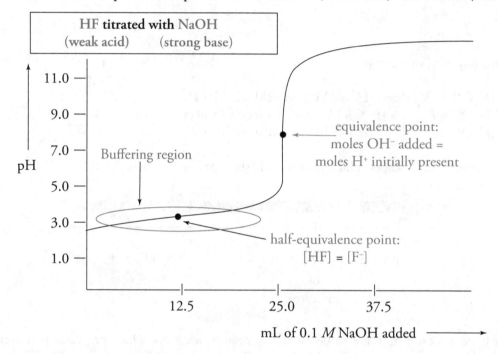

When the amount of titrant added is 0, the pH is of course just the pH of the original, pure solution of HF. Then, as NaOH is added, an equivalent amount of HF will be neutralized according to the reaction

$$NaOH + HF \rightarrow Na^+ + F^- + H_2O$$

As HF is neutralized, the pH will increase. But from the titration curve, we can see that the pH is certainly not increasing very rapidly as we add the first 20 or so mL of NaOH. This should tell you that at the beginning of this titration the solution is behaving as a buffer. As HF is being converted into F^-, we are forming a solution that contains a weak acid and its conjugate base. This section of the titration curve, where the pH changes very gradually, is called the **buffering domain** (or **buffering region**).

Now, as the experiment continues, the solution suddenly loses its buffering capability and the pH increases dramatically. At some point during this drastic increase, all HF is neutralized and no acid remains in solution. Every new ion of OH^- that is added remains in solution. Therefore, the pH continues to increase rapidly until the OH^- concentration in solution is not that much different from the NaOH concentration in the titrant. From here on, the pH doesn't change very much and the curve levels off.

11.10

There is a point during the drastic pH increase at which just enough NaOH has been added to completely neutralize all the HF. This is called the acid-base equivalence point. At this point, we simply have Na^+ ions and F^- ions in solution. Note that the solution should be *basic* here. In fact, from what we know about the behavior of conjugates, we can state the following facts about the equivalence point of different titrations:

- For a weak acid (titrated with a strong base), the equivalence point will occur at a pH > 7.
- For a weak base (titrated with a strong acid), the equivalence point will occur at a pH < 7.
- For a strong acid (titrated with a strong base) or for a strong base (titrated with a strong acid), the equivalence point will occur at pH = 7.

Therefore, by just looking at the pH at the equivalence point of our titration, we can tell whether the acid (or base) we were titrating was weak or strong.

Recall the purpose of this titration experiment: to determine the pK_a (or pK_b) of the unknown weak acid (or weak base). From the titration curve, determine the volume of titrant added at the equivalence point; call it $V_{at\ equiv}$. A key question is this: What's in solution when the volume of added titrant is $1/2\ V_{at\ equiv}$? Let's return to our titration of HF by NaOH. We can read from its titration curve that $V_{at\ equiv} = 25$ mL. When the amount of NaOH added was $1/2\ V_{at\ equiv} = 12.5$ mL, the solution consisted of equal concentrations of HF and F^-, i.e., enough NaOH was added to convert $1/2$ of the HF to F^-. (After all, when the amount of titrant added was twice as much, $V_{at\ equiv} = 25$ mL, *all* of the HF had been converted to F^-. So naturally, when $1/2$ as much was added, only $1/2$ was converted.) Therefore, at this point—called the half-equivalence point—we have

$$[HF]_{at\ half\text{-}equiv} = [F^-]_{at\ half\text{-}equiv}$$

The Henderson-Hasselbalch equation then tells us that

$$pH_{at\ half\text{-}equiv} = pK_a + \log\left(\frac{[F^-]_{at\ half\text{-}equiv}}{[HF]_{at\ half\text{-}equiv}}\right) = pK_a + \log 1 = pK_a$$

The pK_a of HF equals the pH at the half-equivalence point. For our curve, we see that this occurs around pH 3.2, so we conclude that the pK_a of HF is about 3.2.

11.10

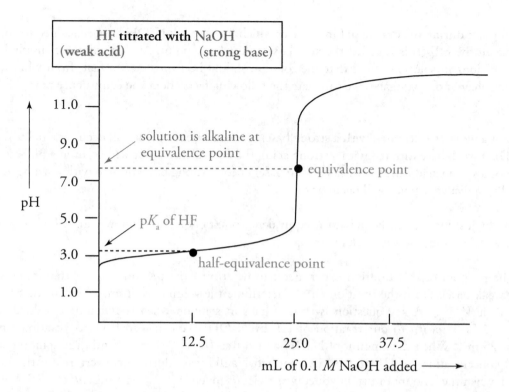

11.10

Compare the sample titration curves for a weak base titrated with a strong acid to the one for a weak acid titrated with a strong base (like the one we just looked at). Note the pH at the equivalence point (relative to pH 7) for each curve.

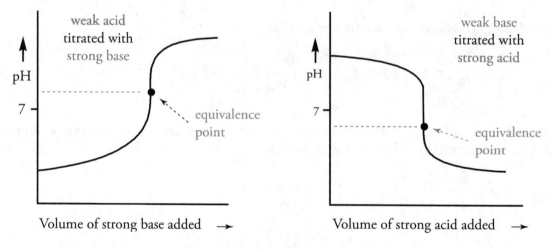

As mentioned above, the titration curve for a strong acid-strong base titration would have the equivalence point at a neutral pH of 7, as shown below.

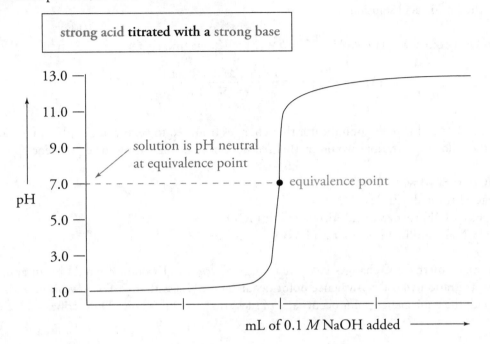

strong acid **titrated with a** strong base

pH

solution is pH neutral
at equivalence point

equivalence point

mL of 0.1 M NaOH added

11.10

The titration curve for the titration of a polyprotic acid (like H_2CO_3 or an amino acid) will have more than one equivalence point. The number of equivalence points is equal to the number of ionizable hydrogens the acid can donate.

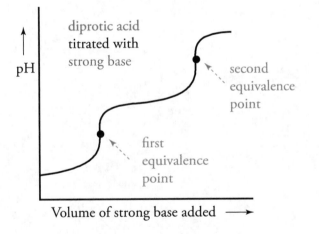

diprotic acid
titrated with
strong base

pH

second
equivalence
point

first
equivalence
point

Volume of strong base added

Example 11-20: A fifty mL solution of HCOOH (formic acid) is titrated with 0.2 M NaOH. The equivalence point is reached when 40 mL of the NaOH solution has been added. What was the original concentration of the formic acid solution?

Solution: Using our formula $a \times [A] \times V_A = b \times [B] \times V_B$, we find that

$$[A] = \frac{b \times [B] \times V_B}{a \times V_A} = \frac{1 \times (0.2\ M) \times (40\ mL)}{1 \times (50\ mL)} = 0.16\ M$$

Example 11-21: Methyl red is an indicator that changes from red to yellow in the pH range 4.4–6.2. For which of the following titrations would methyl red be useful for indicating the equivalence point?

A) HCN titrated with KOH
B) NaOH titrated with HI
C) C_6H_5COOH (benzoic acid) titrated with LiOH
D) $C_6H_5NH_2$ (aniline) titrated with HNO_3

Solution: Since methyl red changes color in a range of *acidic* pH values, it would be an appropriate indicator for a titration whose equivalence point occurs at a pH less than 7. For a weak base titrated with a strong acid, the equivalence point occurs at a pH less than 7. Only choice D describes such a titration.

11.10

Chapter 11 Summary

- Acids are proton donors and electron acceptors; bases are proton acceptors and electron donors.

- Strong acids completely dissociate in water ($K_a > 1$). You should memorize the list of strong acids and bases.

- The higher the K_a (lower the pK_a), the stronger the acid. The higher the K_b (lower the pK_b), the stronger the base.

- For any conjugate acid and base pair, $K_a K_b = K_w$. Therefore, it follows that the stronger the acid, the weaker its conjugate base. Conjugates of strong acids and bases have no acid/base properties in water.

- Amphoteric substances may act as either acids or bases.

- Water is amphoteric, and autoionizes into OH^- and H_3O^+. The equilibrium constant for the autoionization of water is $K_w = [OH^-][H_3O^+]$. At 25°C, $K_w = 1 \times 10^{-14}$.

- $pH = -\log[H_3O^+]$. For a concentration of H_3O^+ given in a 10^{-x} M notation, simply take the negative exponent to find the pH. The same is true for the relationship between $[OH^-]$ and pOH, K_a and pK_a, and K_b and pK_b.

- At 25°C, $pK_a + pK_b = 14$.

- If a salt is dissolved in water and the cation is a stronger acid than water, the resulting solution will have a pH < 7. If the anion is a base stronger than water, the resulting solution will have a pH > 7.

- Buffers resist pH change upon the addition of a small amount of strong acid or base. A higher concentration of buffer resists pH change better than a lower concentration of buffer (that is, the solution has a higher buffering capacity).

- A buffer consists of approximately equal molar amounts of a weak acid and its conjugate base, and maintains a pH close to its pK_a.

- The Henderson-Hasselbalch equation can be used to determine the pH of a buffer solution.

- Indicators are weak acids that change color upon conversion to their conjugate base. An indicator changes color in the range +/– 1 pH unit from its pK_a.

· In a titration, the equivalence point is the point at which all of the original acid or base has been neutralized.

· When a strong acid is titrated against a weak base, the pH at the equivalence point is < 7. When a strong base is titrated against a weak acid, the pH at the equivalence point is > 7. When a strong base is titrated against a strong acid, the pH at the equivalence point is = 7.

· At the half equivalence point of a titration of a weak plus a strong acid or base, the solution has equal concentrations of acid and conjugate base, and pH = pK_a.

CHAPTER 11 FREESTANDING PRACTICE QUESTIONS

1. The pH of a CH_3COOH solution is < 7 because when this compound is added to water:

A) CH_3COOH donates H^+, making $[H^+] > [OH^-]$.
B) CH_3COOH loses OH^-, making $[H^+] < [OH^-]$.
C) CH_3COO^- deprotonates H_2O, increasing $[OH^-]$.
D) CH_3COOH dissociation increases $[H^+]$, thereby increasing K_w.

2. All of the following are amphoteric EXCEPT:

A) HCO_3^-
B) $H_2PO_4^-$
C) SO_4^{2-}
D) $HOOCCOO^-$

3. A graph depicting a titration of a weak acid with a strong base will start at a:

A) high pH and slope downwards with an equivalence pH equal to 7.
B) high pH and slope downwards with an equivalence pH below 7.
C) low pH and slope upwards with an equivalence pH equal to 7.
D) low pH and slope upwards with an equivalence pH above 7.

4. List the following compounds by increasing pK_a:

I. H_2SO_4
II. NH_3
III. CH_3CH_2COOH
IV. HF

A) $I < III < II < IV$
B) $I < IV < III < II$
C) $III < I < IV < II$
D) $II < III < IV < I$

5. The amino and carboxyl terminals of alanine lose protons according to the following equilibrium:

$$^+H_3N - \underset{\underset{CH_3}{|}}{\overset{\overset{H}{|}}{C}} - COOH \; \rightleftharpoons \; ^+H_3N - \underset{\underset{CH_3}{|}}{\overset{\overset{H}{|}}{C}} - COO^- \; \rightleftharpoons \; H_2N - \underset{\underset{CH_3}{|}}{\overset{\overset{H}{|}}{C}} - COO^-$$

Which of the following indicators would be best used to determine the second equivalence point when alanine is titrated with sodium hydroxide?

A) Methyl violet ($pK_b = 13.0$)
B) Methyl yellow ($pK_b = 10.5$)
C) Thymol blue ($pK_b = 12.0$)
D) Phenolphthalein ($pK_b = 4.9$)

6. The K_a of HSCN is equal to 1×10^{-4}. The pH of a HSCN solution:

A) will be approximately 4.
B) will be approximately 10.
C) will increase as [HSCN] increases.
D) cannot be determined from the information given.

7. A 25.0 mL solution of 0.2 M acetic acid ($pK_a = 4.76$) is mixed with 50 mL of 1.0 M sodium acetate ($pK_b = 9.24$). What is the final pH?

A) 4.8
B) 5.8
C) 9.2
D) 10.2

CHAPTER 11 PRACTICE PASSAGE

Blood pH homeostasis is the result of several systems operating within the bloodstream. They collectively maintain blood plasma pH at 7.4, since a drop in pH below 6.8 or rise above 7.8 may result in death.

One component of this system is the enzyme *carbonic anhydrase*, which catalyzes the conversion of CO_2 in the blood to carbonic acid. Carbonic acid, in turn, ionizes to form the carbonic acid-bicarbonate buffer. The interdependence of these reactions is shown below in Equation 1.

$$CO_2(g) + H_2O(l) \rightleftharpoons H_2CO_3(aq) \rightleftharpoons H^+(aq) + HCO_3^-(aq)$$

Equation 1

Uncatalyzed blood CO_2 and H^+ can be found binding to hemoglobin after oxygen liberation in peripheral tissues. As the blood reaches the lungs these actions reverse themselves; hemoglobin binds with oxygen, releasing the CO_2 and H^+ ions. The exchange of gases between the lungs and the blood and other tissues in the body is a physiologic process known as respiration.

A second system, the phosphoric acid buffer, plays a minor role compared to the carbonic acid-bicarbonate buffer. Phosphoric acid (H_3PO_4), the primary reactant of this system, is a triprotic acid, which can ionize three protons. This three-step process is illustrated below:

Reaction	K_a
1 $H_3PO_4(aq) \rightleftharpoons H^+(aq) + H_2PO_4^-(aq)$	$K_{a1} = 7.5 \times 10^{-3}$
2 $H_2PO_4^-(aq) \rightleftharpoons H^+(aq) + HPO_4^{2-}(aq)$	$K_{a2} = 6.2 \times 10^{-8}$
3 $HPO_4^{2-}(aq) \rightleftharpoons H^+(aq) + PO_4^{3-}(aq)$	$K_{a3} = 1.7 \times 10^{-12}$

1. Carbonic acid is best described as:

A) amphoteric.
B) polyprotic.
C) a strong acid.
D) the conjugate acid for CO_2.

2. If CO_2 gas is bubbled continuously in a beaker of water to form carbonic acid, which of the following would be true?

   I. Addition of carbonic anhydrase will increase the K_{eq} of the reaction.
   II. Carbonic acid will increase in concentration until K_{eq} is reached.
   III. Addition of bicarbonate will increase the pH of the system.

A) I only
B) II only
C) III only
D) II and III

3. All of the following statements are true regarding human respiration EXCEPT:

A) when a person's breathing is hampered by conditions such as asthma or emphysema, the blood $[H^+]$ increases.
B) exercise stimulates deeper and more rapid breathing, which increases blood plasma pH.
C) slow, shallow breathing allows CO_2 to accumulate in the blood.
D) hyperventilation can result in the loss of too much CO_2, causing the accumulation of bicarbonate ions.

4. In the dissociation of phosphoric acid, the trend $K_{a1} > K_{a2} > K_{a3}$ is predominantly due to:

A) an equilibrium shift towards the reactants side in Reactions 2 and 3 due to the release of H^+ in Reaction 1.
B) a smaller radius in the H^+ liberated in Reaction 1 compared to that in Reactions 2 and 3.
C) a slower rate of reaction after subsequent ionizations.
D) an increasing influence of the anion after subsequent ionizations.

5. What is the relationship between the K_{a1} value for phosphoric acid and the K_{b1} value for dihydrogen phosphate?

A) K_{a1} and K_{b1} are inversely related through the dissociation constant for water, K_w.

B) K_{a1} and K_{b1} are directly related through the dissociation constant for water, K_w.

C) The K_{a1} is less than the K_{b1}.

D) There is no relationship between K_{a1} and K_{b1}.

6. What would be the pH of a solution made from combining 50 mL of 0.030 M acetic acid ($K_a = 1.8 \times 10^{-5}$) and 10 mL of 0.15 M sodium acetate?

A) pH = 1.6

B) pH = 2.5

C) pH = 3.3

D) pH = 4.7

SOLUTIONS TO CHAPTER 11 FREESTANDING PRACTICE QUESTIONS

1. **A** CH_3COOH is acetic acid, a common organic, carboxylic acid. It will dissociate in water to produce H^+ and CH_3COO^-, eliminating choice B. An acidic solution (pH < 7) has more H^+ ions in solution than OH^- ions, making choice A the best answer. Choice C can be eliminated because if $[OH^-]$ were to increase, the pH of the solution would be greater than 7, rather than less than 7. Choice D can be eliminated because the only thing that changes the value of K_w, or any equilibrium constant, is temperature.

2. **C** An amphoteric substance is one that can act as both an acid and a base. This definition fits choices A, B, and D because they can all donate or accept a proton. Choice C has no protons for donation and cannot be acidic.

3. **D** A graph showing the titration of a weak acid will start at a low pH and slope upwards as the titrant (in this case a strong base) is added. Therefore, choices A and B cannot be true. As the weak acid and titrant (strong base) react, water and salt are formed as products. The salt will determine the pH at the equivalence point. The conjugate acid of a strong base has no acidic properties and will be neutral in solution. However, the conjugate base of the weak acid will be weakly basic. Because of this, the pH at the equivalence point will be above 7.

4. **B** A higher pK_a means a weaker acid, while a lower pK_a means a stronger acid. Since this is a ranking question, start with the extremes. Compound I is a strong acid and will have the lowest pK_a, eliminating choices C and D. Compound II is the only base so it will have the largest pK_a and choice A can be eliminated.

5. **D** Alanine is a neutral amino acid with an isoelectric point close to 7. Therefore, the second equivalence point represents when all the ammonium residue of the zwitterion (the middle structure shown in the question) is deprotonated. This must occur at a basic pH. An appropriate indicator will change color if its pK_a is ±1 of the pH at this equivalence point. Therefore, the desired indicator should have a $pK_a > 7$, or $pK_b < 7$, making choice D the best answer. Another approach to this question is to recognize that no numerical data are provided and choice D is the only indicator for a basic region. There would be no other reasonable way to choose between choices A, B, and C.

6. **D** The K_a of an acid is a measure of its ability to dissociate in water, not the pH of a solution (the smaller the K_a the weaker the acid). If we know the $[H^+]$ of a solution we can find the pH by finding $-\log[H^+]$, but we cannot find the pH of a weak acid solution from only the K_a. We must also know the concentration of the acid. Choice A is a trap answer if you confuse pK_a with pH. The greater the concentration of an acid, the more H^+ ions will be in solution. However, this will *decrease* the pH of the solution, not increase it (choices B and C can be eliminated). By process of elimination, choice D is the best answer.

7. **B** The sodium acetate solution will be completely ionized:

$$NaC_2H_3O_2 \rightarrow Na^+ + C_2H_3O_2^-$$

However, acetic acid will have negligible dissociation in solution:

$$HC_2H_3O_2 \rightleftharpoons H^+ + C_2H_3O_2^- \ (K_a \approx 1\times10^{-5})$$

Therefore, for the combined solution, it is reasonable to assume that all of the $HC_2H_3O_2$ is contributed from the acid solution, and all of the $C_2H_3O_2^-$ is contributed from the salt solution:

$$(0.2 \ M \ HC_2H_3O_2)(0.025 \ L) = 5 \times 10^{-3} \ mol \ HC_2H_3O_2$$

$$(1 \ M \ NaC_2H_3O_2)(0.05 \ L) = 5 \times 10^{-2} \ mol \ C_2H_3O_2^-$$

The new volume of 0.075 L cancels out when solving for the pH using the Henderson-Hasselbalch equation:

$$pH = pK_a + \log\frac{[C_2H_3O_2^-]}{[HC_2H_3O_2]}$$

$$pH = 4.76 + \log\frac{\left(\dfrac{5\times10^{-2} \ mol}{0.075 \ L}\right)}{\left(\dfrac{5\times10^{-3} \ mol}{0.075 \ L}\right)}$$

$$pH = 4.76 + \log(10) = 5.76$$

SOLUTIONS TO CHAPTER 11 PRACTICE PASSAGE

1. **B** Even though the bicarbonate ion is amphoteric and can donate and accept a proton, carbonic acid cannot (eliminate choice A). Choice C is eliminated because carbonic acid is not one of the six strong acids you should know for the MCAT (HI, HBr, HCl, $HClO_4$, H_2SO_4, HNO_3). Choice D is false because carbon dioxide and carbonic acid cannot be a conjugate acid-base pair since they differ by more than one H^+. Choice B is correct because carbonic acid has the ability to donate two protons, making it polyprotic.

2. **D** Addition of a catalyst (such as the enzyme carbonic anhydrase) will simply increase the rate of a reaction. It plays no role in shifting the equilibrium, or changing the equilibrium constant making Item I false (eliminate choice A). As carbon dioxide is bubbled through, carbonic acid will form until its equilibrium concentration is attained, making Item II valid (eliminate choice C). Finally, addition of bicarbonate will shift the carbonic acid equilibrium to the reactant side, consuming H^+ in the process. Since the concentration of H^+ will decrease, pH will increase, making Item III valid (eliminate choice B).

3. **D**   Choices A and C can be eliminated because they create the same effect. A decrease in breathing rate causes less CO_2 to exchange, leading to an increase in CO_2 remaining in the blood (i.e., increased CO_2 concentration). Consequently, this shifts the equilibria shown in Figure 1 to the right, which results in increased H^+ concentration, and decreased pH. Choice B is the opposite effect. Deeper, more rapid breathing expels more CO_2, decreasing the CO_2 in the blood and increasing pH. Hyperventilation may involve the loss of too much CO_2. This loss will shift the equilibria shown in Equation 1 to the left. Loss of bicarbonate ions will result, making choice D the only statement that is NOT true.

4. **D**   Generation of H^+ in Reaction 1 is coupled with a release of $H_2PO_4^-$. Both the product and reactant sides of Reaction 2 are increased proportionally, causing no shift in equilibrium (eliminate choice A). Atomic radius is a function of an atom's position in the periodic table. Thus, the radius of H^+ is the same in all three reactions, eliminating choice B. Equilibrium constants have no relationship to reaction rates, so choice C can be eliminated. The K_a values progressively decrease when removing a proton from a polyprotic acid because it is more difficult to remove a proton from an anion compared to a neutral molecule. In subsequent ionizations, the anion becomes more negative, resulting in greater difficulty liberating a positively charged H^+ ion.

5. **A**   The relationship between the K_a value of an acid and the K_b value of its conjugate base is through the dissociation constant of water, where $K_w = (K_a)(K_b)$. Therefore, the relationship between K_{a1} and K_{b1} is $K_{a1} = K_w/K_{b1}$; an inverse relationship.

6. **D**   The final solution is composed of (50 mL)(0.03 M) = 1.5 mmol of $HC_2H_3O_2$ and (10 mL) (0.15 M) = 1.5 mmol of $NaC_2H_3O_2$ (or 1.5 mmol of $C_2H_3O_2^-$). The total volume will be 60 mL and the starting concentration of acetic acid will be the same as the starting concentration of its conjugate base. Since acetic acid is a weak acid, any subsequent dissociation will be relatively insignificant and the equilibrium concentrations of acid and base will remain approximately the same. When the concentration of the two species in a conjugate pair are equal, the pK_a = pH from the Henderson-Hasselbalch equation: pH = pK_a + log [conjugate base]/[acid]. The pK_a of acetic acid ($K_a = 1.8 \times 10^{-5}$) is approximately 4.7.

Chapter 12
Electrochemistry

Oxidation # = how many e⁻ an atom is donating or accepting

12.1 OXIDATION-REDUCTION REACTIONS

Recall that the **oxidation number** (or **oxidation state**) of each atom in a molecule describes how many electrons it is donating or accepting in the overall bonding of the molecule. Many elements can assume different oxidation states depending on the bonds they make. A reaction in which the oxidation numbers of any of the reactants change is called an **oxidation-reduction** (or **redox**) reaction.

In a redox reaction, atoms gain or lose electrons as new bonds are formed. The total number of electrons does not change, of course; they're just redistributed among the atoms. When an atom loses electrons, its oxidation number increases; this is **oxidation**. When an atom gains electrons, the oxidation number decreases; this is **reduction**. A mnemonic device is helpful:

LEO the lion says GER

LEO: Lose Electrons = Oxidation

GER: Gain Electrons = Reduction

Another popular mnemonic is

OIL RIG

OIL: Oxidation Is electron Loss

RIG: Reduction Is electron Gain

An atom that is oxidized in a reaction loses electrons to another atom. We call the oxidized atom a **reducing agent** or **reductant**, because by giving up electrons, it reduces another atom that gains the electrons. On the other hand, the atom that gains the electrons has been **reduced**. We call the reduced atom an **oxidizing agent** or **oxidant**, because it oxidizes another atom that loses the electrons. (You may want to review Section 3.14 on Oxidation States.)

Example 12-1: In an oxidation-reduction, the oxidation number of an aluminum atom changes from 0 to +3. The aluminum atom has been:

A) reduced, and is a reducing agent.
B) reduced, and is an oxidizing agent.
C) oxidized, and is a reducing agent.
D) oxidized, and is an oxidizing agent.

Solution: Since the oxidation number has increased, the atom's been oxidized. And since it's been oxidized, it reduced something else and thus acted as a reducing agent. Therefore, the answer is C.

Take a look at this redox reaction:

$$Fe + 2\ HCl \rightarrow FeCl_2 + H_2$$

The oxidation state of iron changes from 0 to +2. The oxidation state of hydrogen changes from +1 to 0. (The oxidation state of chlorine remains at −1.) So, iron has lost two electrons, and two protons (H^+) have gained one electron each. Therefore, the iron has been oxidized, and the hydrogens have been reduced. In order to better see the exchange of electrons, a redox reaction can be broken down into a pair of **half-reactions** that show the oxidation and reduction separately. These **ion-electron** equations show only the actual oxidized or reduced species—and the electrons involved—in an electron-balanced reaction. For the redox reaction shown above, the ion-electron half-reactions are:

$$\text{oxidation:} \quad Fe \rightarrow Fe^{2+} + 2e^-$$
$$\text{reduction:} \quad 2\,H^+ + 2e^- \rightarrow H_2$$

Example 12-2: For the redox reaction

$$3\,MnO_2 + 2\,Al \rightarrow 2\,Al_2O_3 + 3\,Mn$$

which of the following shows the oxidation half-reaction?

A) $Mn^{4+} + 4e^- \rightarrow Mn$
B) $Mn^{2+} + 2e^- \rightarrow Mn$
C) $Al \rightarrow Al^{3+} + 3e^-$
D) $Al^{4+} \rightarrow Al^{6+} + 6e^-$

Solution: First, eliminate choices A and B since they're *reduction* half-reactions. We can then eliminate choice D for two reasons: First, Al^{4+} is not the species of aluminum on the reactant side; second, it's not balanced electrically. The answer must be C.

12.2 GALVANIC CELLS

Because a redox reaction involves the transfer of electrons, and the flow of electrons constitutes an electric current that can do work, we can use a spontaneous redox reaction to generate an electric current. A device for doing this is called a **galvanic** (or **voltaic**) **cell**, the main features of which are shown in the figure below.

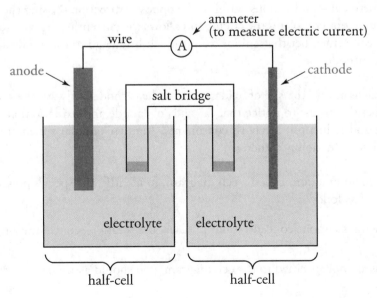

One **electrode**, generally composed of a metal (labeled the **anode**) gets oxidized, and the electrons its atoms lose travel along the wire to a second metal electrode (labeled the **cathode**). It is at the cathode that reduction takes place. In this way, the anode acts as an electron source, while the cathode acts as an electron sink. Electrons always flow through the conducting wire from the anode to the cathode. This electron flow is the electric current that is produced by the spontaneous redox reaction between the electrodes.

Let's look at a specific galvanic cell, with the anode made of zinc, and the cathode made of copper. The anode is immersed in a $ZnSO_4$ solution, the cathode is immersed in a $CuSO_4$ solution, and the half cells are connected by a **salt bridge** containing an aqueous solution of KNO_3. When the electrodes are connected by a wire, zinc atoms in the anode are oxidized ($Zn \rightarrow Zn^{2+} + 2e^-$), and the electrons travel through the wire to the cathode. There, the Cu^{2+} ions in solution pick up these electrons and get reduced to copper metal ($Cu^{2+} + 2e^- \rightarrow Cu$), which accumulates on the copper cathode. The sulfate anions balance the charge on the Zn^{2+}, but do not participate in any redox reaction, and are therefore known as spectator ions.

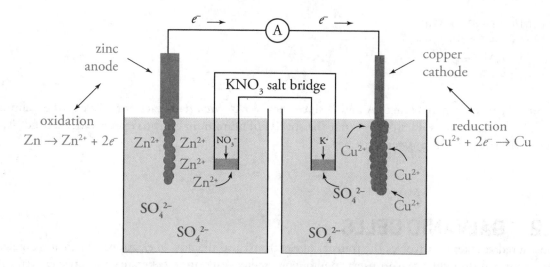

The Zn^{2+} ions that remain in the solution in the zinc half-cell attract NO_3^- ions from the salt bridge, and K^+ ions in the salt bridge are attracted into the copper half-cell. Notice that anions in solution travel from the right cell to the left cell—and cations travel in the opposite direction—using the salt bridge as a conduit. This movement of ions completes the circuit and allows the current in the wire to continue, until the zinc strip is consumed. Remember that anions from the salt bridge go to the anode and cations from the salt bridge go to the cathode.

Notice that the anode is always the site of oxidation, and the cathode is always the site of reduction. One way to help remember this is just to notice that "a" and "o" (anode and oxidation) are both vowels, while "c" and "r" (cathode and reduction) are both consonants. Another popular mnemonic is "an ox, red cat" for "anode = oxidation, reduction = cathode."

We often use a shorthand notation, called a **cell diagram**, to identify the species present in a galvanic cell. Cell diagrams are read as follows:

Anode | Anodic solution (concentration) || Cathodic solution (concentration) | Cathode

If the concentrations are not specified in the cell diagram, you should assume they are 1 M.

Example 12-3: In the electrochemical cell described by the following cell diagram, what reaction occurs at the anode?

$$\text{Zn}(s) \mid \text{Zn}^{2+}(aq) \mid\mid \text{Cl}^-(aq) \mid \text{Cl}_2(g)$$

A) $\text{Zn} \rightarrow \text{Zn}^{2+} + 2e^-$
B) $\text{Zn}^{2+} + 2e^- \rightarrow \text{Zn}$
C) $2\,\text{Cl}^- \rightarrow \text{Cl}_2 + 2e^-$
D) $\text{Cl}_2 + 2e^- \rightarrow 2\,\text{Cl}^-$

Solution: For any electrochemical cell, oxidation occurs at the anode, and reduction occurs at the cathode. Therefore, we're looking for an oxidation, and choices B and D are eliminated. Since Zn is present at the anode, the answer is A.

Example 12-4: In the absence of a salt bridge, charge separation develops. The anode develops a positive charge and the cathode develops a negative charge, quickly halting the flow of electrons. In this state, the battery resembles:

A) a resistor.
B) a capacitor.
C) a transformer.
D) an inductor.

Solution: The question tells us that the result of removing a salt bridge is charge separation. In physics, we learned that a capacitor is a device that stores electrical energy due to the separation of charge on adjacent surfaces. Thus, choice B is the correct choice.

12.3 STANDARD REDUCTION POTENTIALS

To determine whether the redox reaction of a cell is spontaneous and can produce an electric current, we need to figure out the cell voltage. Each half-reaction has a potential (E), which is the cell voltage it would have if the other electrode were the standard reference electrode. (*Note*: We usually consider cells at standard conditions: 25°C, 1 atm pressure, aqueous solutions at 1 M concentrations, and with substances in their standard states. To indicate standard conditions, we use a ° superscript on quantities such as E and ΔG.) By definition, the standard reference electrode is the site of the redox reaction $2\,\text{H}^+ + 2e^- \rightarrow \text{H}_2$, which is assigned a potential of 0.00 volts. By adding the half-reaction potential for a given pair of electrodes, we get the cell's overall voltage. Tables of half-reaction potentials are usually given for reductions only. Since each cell has a reduction half-reaction and an oxidation half-reaction, we get the potential of the oxidation by simply reversing the sign of the corresponding reduction potential.

For example, the standard reduction potential for the half-reaction $\text{Cu}^{2+} + 2e^- \rightarrow \text{Cu}$ is $+0.34$ V. The standard reduction potential for the half-reaction $\text{Zn}^{2+} + 2e^- \rightarrow \text{Zn}$ is -0.76 V. Reversing the zinc reduction to an oxidation, we get $Zn \rightarrow Zn^{2+} + 2e^-$, with a potential of +0.76 V. Therefore, the overall cell voltage for the zinc-copper cell is (+0.76 V) + (+0.34 V) = +1.10 V:

oxidation:	$Zn \rightarrow Zn^{2+} + 2e^-$	$E° = +0.76$ V
reduction:	$Cu^{2+} + 2e^- \rightarrow Cu$	$E° = +0.34$ V
	$Zn + Cu^{2+} \rightarrow Zn^{2+} + Cu$	$E° = +1.10$ V

The free-energy change, $\Delta G°$, for a redox reaction in which cell voltage is $E°$ is given by the equation

$$\Delta G° = -nFE°$$

where n is the number of moles of electrons transferred and F stands for a **faraday** (the magnitude of the charge of one mole of electrons, approximately 96,500 coulombs). Since a reaction is spontaneous if $\Delta G°$ is negative, this equation tells us that the redox reaction in a cell will be spontaneous if the cell voltage is positive. Since the cell voltage for our zinc-copper cell was +1.10 V, we know the reaction will be spontaneous and produce an electric current that can do work.

> If the cell voltage is positive, then the reaction is spontaneous.
>
> If the cell voltage is negative, then the reaction is nonspontaneous.

Let's do another example and consider what would happen if the zinc electrode in our cell above were replaced by a gold electrode, given that the **standard reduction potential** for the reaction $Au^{3+} + 3e^- \rightarrow Au$ is $E° = +1.50$ V. The redox reaction that we're investigating is

$$Au + Cu^{2+} \rightarrow Au^{3+} + Cu$$

Let's first break this down into half-reactions:

$Au \rightarrow Au^{3+} + 3e^-$	$E° = -1.50$ V
$Cu^{2+} + 2e^- \rightarrow Cu$	$E° = +0.34$ V

The overall reaction is not electron balanced; but by multiplying the first half-reaction by 2 and the second half-reaction by 3, we get

$2\,Au \rightarrow 2\,Au^{3+} + 6e^-$	$E° = -1.50$ V
$3\,Cu^{2+} + 6e^- \rightarrow 3\,Cu$	$E° = +0.34$ V
$2\,Au + 3\,Cu^{2+} \rightarrow 2\,Au^{3+} + 3\,Cu$	$E° = -1.16$ V

The final equation is now electron balanced. Notice that although we multiplied the half-reactions by stoichiometric coefficients, we did *not* multiply the potentials by those coefficients. You never multiply the potential by a coefficient, even if you multiply a half-reaction by a coefficient to get the balanced equation for the reaction. This is because the potentials are *intrinsic* to the identities of the species involved and do not depend on the number of moles of the species.

Because the cell voltage is negative, this reaction would not be spontaneous. However, it would be spontaneous in the other direction; that is, if copper were the *anode* and gold the *cathode*, then the potential of the cell would be +1.16 V, which implies a spontaneous reaction.

Oxidizing and Reducing Agents

We can also use reduction potentials to determine whether reactants are good or poor oxidizing or reducing agents. For example, let's look again at the half-reactions in our original zinc-copper cell. The half-reaction $Zn^{2+} + 2e^- \rightarrow Zn$ has a standard potential of -0.76 V, and the half-reaction $Cu^{2+} + 2e^- \rightarrow Cu$ has a standard potential of $+0.34$ V. The fact that the reduction of Zn^{2+} is nonspontaneous means that the oxidation of Zn is spontaneous, so Zn would rather give up electrons. If it does, this means that Zn acts as a reducing agent because in giving up electrons it reduces something else. The fact that the reduction of Cu^{2+} has a positive potential tells us that this reaction would be spontaneous at standard conditions. In other words, Cu^{2+} is a good oxidizing agent because it's looking to accept electrons, thereby oxidizing something else. So, in general, if a reduction half-reaction has a large negative potential, then the product is a good reducing agent. On the other hand, if a reduction half-reaction has a large positive potential, then the reactant is a good oxidizing agent. Now, whether something is a "good" oxidizing or reducing agent depends on what it's being compared to. So, to be more precise, we should say this:

> The more negative the reduction potential, the weaker the reactant is as an oxidizing agent, and the stronger the product is as a reducing agent.
>
> The more positive the reduction potential, the stronger the reactant is as an oxidizing agent, and the weaker the product is as a reducing agent.

For example, given that $Pb^{2+} + 2e^- \rightarrow Pb$ has a standard potential of -0.13 V, and $Al^{3+} + 3e^- \rightarrow Al$ has a standard potential of -1.67 V, what could we conclude? Well, since Al^{3+} has a large negative reduction potential, the product, aluminum metal, is a good reducing agent. In fact, because the reduction potential of Al^{3+} is more negative than that of Pb^{2+}, we'd say that aluminum is a stronger reducing agent than lead.

Example 12-5: A galvanic cell is set to operate at standard conditions. If one electrode is made of magnesium and the other is made of copper, then the magnesium electrode will serve as the:

A)   anode and be the site of oxidation.
B)   anode and be the site of reduction.
C)   cathode and be the site of oxidation.
D)   cathode and be the site of reduction.

Solution: First, eliminate choices B and C since the anode is always the site of oxidation and the cathode is always the site of reduction. From the table, we see that the reduction of Mg^{2+} is nonspontaneous, whereas the reduction of Cu^{2+} is spontaneous.

Reaction	$E°$ (volts)
$Li^+ + e^- \rightarrow Li$	-3.05
$Mg^{2+} + 2e^- \rightarrow Mg$	-2.36
$Al^{3+} + 3e^- \rightarrow Al$	-1.67
$Zn^{2+} + 2e^- \rightarrow Zn$	-0.76
$Fe^{2+} + 2e^- \rightarrow Fe$	-0.44
$Pb^{2+} + 2e^- \rightarrow Pb$	-0.13
$2 H^+ + 2e^- \rightarrow H_2$	0.00
$Cu^{2+} + 2e^- \rightarrow Cu$	0.34
$Ag^+ + e^- \rightarrow Ag$	0.80
$Pd^{2+} + 2e^- \rightarrow Pd$	0.99
$Pt^{2+} + 2e^- \rightarrow Pt$	1.20
$Au^{3+} + 3e^- \rightarrow Au$	1.50
$F_2 + 2e^- \rightarrow 2 F^-$	2.87

Therefore, the copper electrode will serve as the cathode and be the site of reduction, and the magnesium electrode will serve as the anode and be the site of oxidation (choice A).

Example 12-6: What is the standard cell voltage for the reduction of Ag^+ by Al?

Solution: The half-reactions are

$$Ag^+ + e^- \rightarrow Ag \qquad E° = 0.80 \text{ V}$$
$$Al \rightarrow Al^{3+} + 3e^- \qquad E° = +1.67 \text{ V}$$

Although we'd multiply both sides of the first half-reaction by the stoichiometric coefficient 3 before adding it to the second one to give the overall, electron-balanced redox reaction, we don't bother to do that here. The question is asking only for $E°$, and the potentials of the half-reactions are not affected by stoichiometric coefficients. Adding the potentials of these half-reactions gives us the overall cell voltage: $E° = 2.47$ V.

Example 12-7: For the reaction below, which of the following statements is true?

$$2 \text{ Au} + 3 \text{ Fe}^{2+} \rightarrow 2 \text{ Au}^{3+} + 3 \text{ Fe}$$

A) The reaction is spontaneous, because its cell voltage is positive.
B) The reaction is spontaneous, because its cell voltage is negative.
C) The reaction is not spontaneous, because its cell voltage is positive.
D) The reaction is not spontaneous, because its cell voltage is negative.

Solution: First, eliminate choices B and C. Even without looking at the table of reduction potentials, these choices can't be correct. If the cell voltage $E°$ is negative, then the reaction is nonspontaneous, and if $E°$ is positive, then the reaction is spontaneous. The half-reactions are

$$2(\text{Au} \rightarrow \text{Au}^{3+} + 3e^-) \qquad E° = -1.50 \text{ V}$$
$$3(\text{Fe}^{2+} + 2e^- \rightarrow \text{Fe}) \qquad E° = -0.44 \text{ V}$$

Notice again that the question is really asking only about $E°$, and the potentials of the half-reactions are *not* affected by stoichiometric coefficients (2 and 3, in this case). Since each of these half-reactions has a negative value for $E°$, the cell voltage (obtained by adding them) will also be negative, so the answer is D.

Example 12-8: Of the following, which is the strongest reducing agent?

A) Zn
B) Fe
C) Pd
D) Pd^{2+}

Solution: Remember the rule: The more negative the reduction potential, the stronger the product is as a reducing agent. Zn (choice A) is the product of a redox half-reaction whose potential is −0.76 V. Fe (choice B) is the product of a redox half-reaction whose potential is −0.44 V. So, we know we can eliminate choice B. Pd (choice C) is the product of a redox half-reaction whose potential is +0.99 V, so C is eliminated. Finally, in order for Pd^{2+} to be a reducing agent, it would have to be oxidized—that is, lose more electrons. A cation getting further oxidized? Not likely, especially when there's a neutral metal (choice A) that is happier to do so.

Example 12-9: Of the following, which is the strongest oxidizing agent?

A) Al^{3+}
B) Ag^+
C) Au^{3+}
D) Cu^{2+}

Solution: Remember the rule: The more positive the reduction potential, the stronger the reactant is as an oxidizing agent. Al^{3+} (choice A) is the reactant of a redox half-reaction whose potential is negative, so we can probably eliminate choice A right away. Ag^+ (choice B) is the reactant of a redox half-reaction whose potential is +0.80 V. (Now we know that A can be eliminated). Au^{3+} (choice C) is the reactant of a redox half-reaction whose potential is +1.50 V, so now B is eliminated. Finally, Cu^{2+} (choice D) is the reactant of a redox half-reaction whose potential is only +0.34 V, so choice C is better.

Example 12-10: Which of the following best approximates the value of $\Delta G°$ for this reaction:

$$2\,Al + 3\,Cu^{2+} \rightarrow 2\,Al^{3+} + 3\,Cu?$$

A) $-(12)(96{,}500)$ J
B) $-(6)(96{,}500)$ J
C) $+(6)(96{,}500)$ J
D) $+(12)(96{,}500)$ J

Solution: The half-reactions are

$$2(Al \rightarrow Al^{3+} + 3e^-) \qquad E° = +1.67 \text{ V}$$
$$3(Cu^{2+} + 2e^- \rightarrow Cu) \qquad E° = 0.34 \text{ V}$$

so the overall cell voltage is $E° = 2.01$ V ≈ 2 V. Because the number of electrons transferred is $n = 2 \times 3 = 6$, the equation $\Delta G° = -nFE°$ tells us that choice A is the answer:

$$\Delta G° = -(6)(96{,}500)(2) \text{ J} = -(12)(96{,}500) \text{ J}$$

12.4 NONSTANDARD CONDITIONS

All the previous discussion of potentials assumed the conditions to be standard state, meaning that all aqueous reactants in the mixture were 1 M in concentration. So long as this is true, the tabulated values for reduction potentials apply to each half reaction.

However, since conditions are not always standard we must have a way to alternatively, and more generally, describe the voltage of an electrochemical reaction. To do this we use the Nernst equation.

Recall the following relationship:

$$\Delta G = \Delta G° + RT \ln Q$$

If we substitute ΔG and $\Delta G°$ with their respective relation to E and $E°$, we arrive at

$$-nFE = -nFE° + RT \ln Q$$

or

$$E = E° - \left(\frac{RT}{nF}\right) \ln Q$$

This is the **Nernst equation**. It describes how deviations in temperature and concentration of reactants can alter the voltage of a reaction under nonstandard conditions. As in the standard chemical systems previously discussed, the concentrations of product and reactants will change until $Q = K_{eq}$, and $E = 0$.

Concentration Cells

A **concentration cell** is a galvanic cell that has identical electrodes but which has half-cells with different ion concentrations. Since the electrodes and relevant ions in the two beakers have the same identities, the *standard* cell voltage, $E°$, would be zero. But, such a cell is *not* standard because both electrolytic solutions in the half-cells are not 1 M. So even though the electrodes are the same, in a concentration cell there *will* be a potential difference between them, and an electric current will be produced. For example, let's say both electrodes are made of zinc, and the $[Zn^{2+}]$ concentrations in the electrolytes were 0.1 M and 0.3 M, respectively. We'd expect electrons to be induced to flow through the conducting wire to the half-cell with the higher concentration of these positive ions. So, the zinc electrode in the 0.1 M solution would serve as the anode, with the liberated electrons flowing across the wire to the zinc electrode in the 0.3 M solution, which serves as the cathode. When the concentrations of the solutions become equal, the reaction will stop.

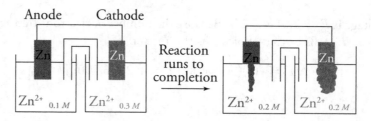

12.5 REDOX TITRATIONS

Just as the titration of an acid with a strong base of known concentration can provide information about the initial acid solution (most notably the concentration and pK_a), titration of a redox active species with a strong oxidant or reductant can be used to determine similar unknowns.

Most redox titrations involve the use of a redox indicator. Much like an indicator in acid/base chemistry, a redox indicator uses a change in color to determine the **endpoint**. However, in a redox reaction, this change in color is due to a change in oxidation state rather than loss or gain of a proton. One commonly used redox indicator is the Ce^{4+} ion, a strong oxidant according to the equation below:

$$Ce^{4+} \ + \ 1e^- \ \rightarrow \ Ce^{3+} \qquad E^0 \approx 1.5 \text{ V (1 } M \text{ HCl solution)}$$

The Ce^{4+} ion is bright yellow in solution, whereas the reduced Ce^{3+} is colorless. This color change, along with the comparatively high redox potential, make Ce^{4+} an ideal indicator for the determination of the concentration of solutions of oxidizable species.

For example, cerium is known to oxidize secondary alcohols to ketones in aqueous solution. As such, titration with Ce^{4+} is an appropriate method for the determination of alcohol concentration in solution, or for the determination of the number of secondary hydroxyl groups present in a chemical species. As long as the Ce^{4+} added to the solution is consumed, the solution will remain colorless. However, the solution will turn yellow immediately after all oxidizable hydroxyls have been consumed. Knowledge of the concentration of the Ce^{4+} titrant allows for the determination of initial alcohol concentration.

A redox titration curve, similar to an acid-base titration curve, can be plotted for any such redox titration. An example is given below where a generic reductant is titrated with Ce^{4+}.

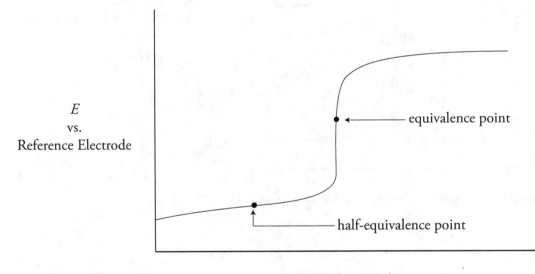

E
vs.
Reference Electrode

equivalence point

half-equivalence point

Volume Ce^{4+}

The equivalence point on the plot above will coincide with the solution turning yellow, indicating the completion of the redox reaction and the total consumption of the reductant as described by the system's balanced redox equation. The significance of the half-equivalence point can be seen in the Nernst equation:

$$E = E° - (RT/nF) \ln Q$$

In this case, Q refers to the ratio of oxidized and non-oxidized reactant. At the half-equivalence point these two quantities are equal and $Q = 1$. Since $\ln(1) = 0$, at the half equivalence point the value of E (measured against whichever reference electrode one chooses) is equal to the value of $E°$ for the redox couple being titrated.

12.6 ELECTROLYTIC CELLS

Unlike a galvanic cell, an **electrolytic cell** *uses* an external voltage source (such as a battery) to *create an electric current* that forces a nonspontaneous redox reaction to occur. This is known as **electrolysis**. A typical example of an electrolytic cell is one used to form sodium metal and chlorine gas from molten NaCl.

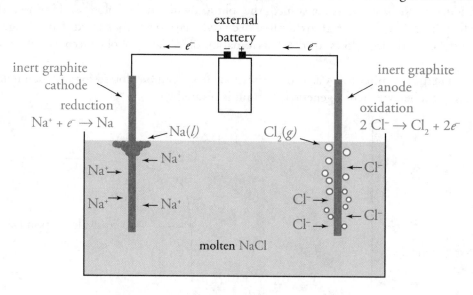

The half-reactions for converting molten Na^+Cl^- into sodium and chlorine are:

$$Na^+ + e^- \rightarrow Na(l) \qquad E° = -2.71 \text{ V}$$
$$2 Cl^- \rightarrow Cl_2(g) + 2e^- \qquad E° = -1.36 \text{ V}$$

The standard voltage for the overall reaction is −4.07 V, which means the reaction is *not* spontaneous. The electrolytic cell shown above uses an external battery to remove electrons from chloride ions and forces sodium ions to accept them. In so doing, the sodium ions are reduced to sodium metal, and the chloride ions are oxidized to produce chlorine gas, which bubbles out of the electrolyte.

Electrolytic cells are also used for plating a thin layer of metal on top of another material, a process known as **electroplating**. If a fork is used as the cathode in an electrolytic cell whose electrolyte contains silver ions, silver will precipitate onto the fork, producing a silver-plated fork. Other examples of metal plating include gold-plated jewelry, and plating tin or chromium onto steel (for tin cans and car bumpers).

Galvanic vs. Electrolytic Cells

Notice that in both galvanic cells and electrolytic cells, the anode is the site of oxidation and the cathode is the site of reduction. Furthermore, electrons in the external circuit always move from the anode to the cathode. The difference, of course, is that a galvanic cell uses a spontaneous redox reaction to create an electric current, whereas an electrolytic cell uses an electric current to force a nonspontaneous redox reaction to occur.

It follows that in a galvanic cell, the anode is negative and the cathode is positive since electrons are spontaneously moving from a negative to a positive charge. However, in an electrolytic cell the anode is positive and the cathode is negative since electrons are being forced to move where they don't want to go.

Galvanic	Electrolytic
Reduction at cathode	
Oxidation at anode	
Electrons flow from anode to cathode	
Anions migrate to anode	
Cations migrate to cathode	
Spontaneously generates electrical power ($\Delta G° < 0$)	Nonspontaneous, requires an external electric power source ($\Delta G° > 0$)
Total $E°$ of reaction is positive	Total $E°$ of reaction is negative
Anode is negative	Anode is positive
Cathode is positive	Cathode is negative

Example 12-11: The final products of the electrolysis of aqueous NaCl are most likely:

A) Na(*s*) and Cl$_2$(*g*)
B) HOCl(*aq*) and Na(*s*)
C) Na(*s*) and O$_2$(*g*)
D) NaOH(*aq*) and HOCl(*aq*)

Solution: This is a little tricky, but it provides a good example of using the process of elimination. We're not expected to be able to answer this question outright, since there is virtually no information provided. Instead, realize that choices A, B and C list metallic sodium as a final product. That's a problem because we're in an aqueous medium, and we know that sodium metal reacts violently in water to form NaOH and hydrogen gas and fire. So after eliminating these choices, we're left with choice D.

Common Rechargeable Batteries

One particularly useful galvanic cell uses two different oxidations states of Pb for its constitutive electrodes and sulfuric acid as an electrolyte. Often referred to as lead-acid batteries, these cells constitute the oldest type of rechargeable batteries, and are perhaps most commonly employed as automobile batteries.

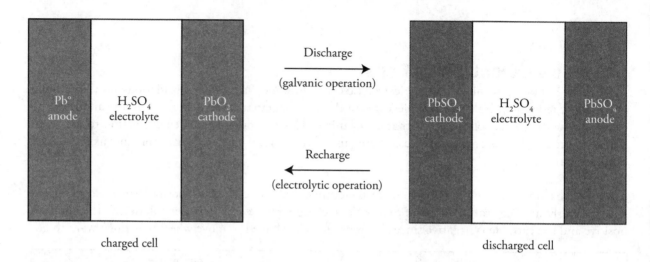

As depicted in the simplified figure above, fully charged lead acid batteries utilize Pb° as an anodic electrode and a cathode consisting of PbO_2. As the battery discharges, Pb° undergoes a two-electron oxidation to $PbSO_4$, while PbO_2 is reduced to the same species, as described by the following equations.

$$Pb^\circ + HSO_4^- \rightarrow PbSO_4 + H^+ + 2e^-$$

$$PbO_2 + HSO_4^- + 3\,H^+ + 2e^- \rightarrow PbSO_4 + 2\,H_2O$$

Recharging the battery involves reversing the electron flow of discharge with applied voltage, as an electrolytic cell. The oxidation of $PbSO_4$ back to PbO_2, along with the regeneration of Pb° by the reduction of $PbSO_4$ restores the initial potential of the cell.

Nickel-cadmium batteries, or NiCad batteries, are another common type of rechargeable battery. These cells utilize a metallic Cd° anode and a nickel oxide hydroxide (NiO(OH)) cathode. The redox reactions involved in the discharge of the battery are given below. To facilitate these reactions, NiCad cells contain an alkaline KOH electrolyte.

$$Cd^\circ + 2\,OH^- \rightarrow Cd(OH)_2 + 2e^-$$

$$2\,NiO(OH) + 2\,H_2O + 2e^- \rightarrow 2\,Ni(OH)_2 + 2\,OH^-$$

Recharging spent NiCad batteries, as one might expect, involves applying a voltage to run these two reactions in reverse (typical electrolytic-cell behavior).

12.7 FARADAY'S LAW OF ELECTROLYSIS

We can determine the amounts of sodium metal and chlorine gas produced at the electrodes in the electrolytic cell shown in Section 12.6 using Faraday's law of electrolysis:

> ### Faraday's Law of Electrolysis
> The amount of chemical change is proportional to the amount of electricity that flows through the cell.

For example, let's answer this question: If 5 amps of current flowed in the NaCl electrolytic cell for 1930 seconds, how much sodium metal and chlorine gas would be produced?

Step 1:   First determine the amount of electricity (in coulombs, C) that flowed through the cell.
We use the equation $Q = It$ (that is, charge = current × time) to find that

$$Q = (5 \text{ amps})(1930 \text{ sec}) = 9650 \text{ coulombs}$$

Step 2:   Use the faraday, F, to convert Q from Step 1 to moles of electrons.
The faraday is the magnitude of the charge on 1 mole of electrons; it's a constant equal to $(1.6 \times 10^{-19} \text{ C}/e^-)(6.02 \times 10^{23} \text{ } e^-/\text{mol}) \approx 96{,}500 \text{ C/mol}$. So, if 9650 C of charge flowed through the cell, this represents

$$9650 \text{ C} \times \frac{1 \text{ mol } e^-}{96{,}500 \text{ C}} = 0.1 \text{ mol } e^-$$

Step 3:   Use the stoichiometry of the half-reactions to finish the calculation.
  a)   From the stoichiometry of the reaction $Na^+ + e^- \rightarrow Na$, we see that 1 mole of electrons would give 1 mole of Na. Therefore, 0.1 mol of electrons gives 0.1 mol of Na. Since the molar mass of sodium is 23 g/mol, we'd get $(0.1)(23 \text{ g}) = 2.3$ g of sodium metal deposited onto the cathode.
  b)   From the stoichiometry of the reaction $2 \text{ Cl}^- \rightarrow Cl_2(g) + 2e^-$, we see that for every 1 mole of electrons lost, we get 0.5 mole of $Cl_2(g)$. Since Step 2 told us that 0.1 mol of electrons were liberated at the anode, 0.05 mol of $Cl_2(g)$ was produced. Because the molar mass of Cl_2 is $2(35.5 \text{ g/mol}) = 71$ g/mol, we'd get $(0.05 \text{ mol})(71 \text{ g/mol}) = 3.55$ g of chlorine gas.

Example 12-12: A piece of steel is the cathode in a hot solution of chromic acid (H_2CrO_4) to electroplate it with chromium metal. How much chromium would be deposited onto the steel after 48,250 C of electricity was forced through the cell?

A) $\frac{1}{12}$ mol

B) $\frac{1}{6}$ mol

C) $\frac{1}{4}$ mol

D)   3 mol

Solution: First, we notice that 48,250 C of electricity is equal to $\frac{1}{2}$ faraday (F = 96,500 C/mol). This is equivalent to $\frac{1}{2}$ mole of electrons. In the molecule H_2CrO_4, chromium is in a +6 oxidation state. So, from the stoichiometry of the reaction $Cr^{6+} + 6e^- \rightarrow Cr$, we see that for every 6 moles of electrons gained, we get 1 mole of Cr metal. Another way of looking at this is to say that for every 1 mole of electrons gained, we get just $\frac{1}{6}$ mole of Cr metal. Therefore, if we have a supply of $\frac{1}{2}$ mol of electrons, we'll produce $(\frac{1}{6})(\frac{1}{2}) = \frac{1}{12}$ mol of Cr, choice A.

Chapter 12 Summary

- Oxidation is electron loss; reduction is electron gain (remember "OIL RIG").

- A species that is oxidized is a reducing agent, and a species that is reduced is an oxidizing agent.

- In all electrochemical cells, oxidation occurs at the anode and reduction occurs at the cathode.

- Electrons always flow from the anode to the cathode.

- Salt bridge anions always migrate toward the anode, and cations always migrate toward the cathode.

- The free energy of an electrochemical cell can be calculated from its potential based on $\Delta G° = -nFE°$.

- A galvanic cell spontaneously generates electrical power $(-\Delta G, +E)$.

- An electrolytic cell consists of nonspontaneous reactions and requires an external electrical power source $(+\Delta G, -E)$.

- In a galvanic cell, electrons spontaneously flow from the negative $(-)$ terminal to the positive $(+)$ terminal. Therefore, it follows that in a galvanic cell the anode is negatively charged $(-)$ and the cathode is positively charged $(+)$.

- In an electrolytic cell, electrons are forced from the positive $(+)$ terminal to the negative $(-)$ terminal, and therefore the anode is positively charged $(+)$ and the cathode is negatively charged $(-)$.

- Standard reduction and oxidation potentials are intrinsic values and therefore should not be multiplied by molar coefficients in balanced half reactions.

- For a given reduction potential, the reverse reaction, or oxidation potential, has the same magnitude of E but the opposite sign.

- Faraday's law of electrolysis states that the amount of chemical change is proportional to the amount of electricity that flows through the cell.

- Under nonstandard conditions, the potential of an electrochemical cell can be calculated using the Nernst equation: $E = E° - (\frac{RT}{nF})\ln Q$.

CHAPTER 12 FREESTANDING PRACTICE QUESTIONS

1. Typical dry cell batteries contain a zinc anode and a carbon cathode and produce a potential difference of 1.5 V. Given that many electronic devices require additional voltage, which of the following would result in an overall increase in voltage?

    I.   Doubling the quantity of $Zn(s)$
    II. Placing two batteries in parallel
    III. Replacing $Zn(s)$ with $Na(s)$

A) I only
B) III only
C) I and II only
D) II and III only

2. Given the following reactions:

$$Pb^{2+} + 2e^- \rightarrow Pb(s) \quad E° = -0.13 \text{ V}$$
$$Fe(s) \rightarrow Fe^{2+} + 2e^- \quad E° = 0.45 \text{ V}$$

Which one of the following is true?

A) $Pb(s)$ is a better reductant than $Fe(s)$
B) $Fe(s)$ is a worse reductant than $Pb(s)$
C) Fe^{2+} is a better oxidant than Pb^{2+}
D) Pb^{2+} is a better oxidant than Fe^{2+}

3. Which of the following best characterizes the spontaneous half-reaction below under standard conditions?

$$Pd^{2+} + 2e^- \rightarrow Pd$$

A) $\Delta G° > 0$ and $E° < 0$
B) $\Delta G° < 0$ and $E° < 0$
C) $\Delta G° > 0$ and $E° > 0$
D) $\Delta G° < 0$ and $E° > 0$

4. High valent metals (those with large, positive oxidation states) are often used as strong oxidizing agents. Which of the following compounds would have the most positive reduction potential vs. a standard hydrogen electrode?

A) $FeCl_3$
B) OsO_4
C) $Zn(NO_3)Cl$
D) $W(CO)_6$

5. Which of the following best describes the difference between a galvanic cell and an electrolytic cell?

A) In a galvanic cell, the anode is the site of oxidation, whereas in an electrolytic cell the anode is the site of reduction.
B) In a galvanic cell, the cathode is the negative electrode, whereas in an electrolytic cell the cathode is the positive electrode.
C) In a galvanic cell, spontaneous reactions generate a current, whereas in an electrolytic cell a current forces nonspontaneous reactions to occur.
D) In a galvanic cell, the electrons flow from anode to cathode, whereas in an electrolytic cell the electrons flow from cathode to anode.

6. To give "white gold" a white appearance, it is plated with rhodium by immersion in a rhodium sulfate solution $(Rh_2(SO_4)_3(aq))$. Provided with a current of 2.0 A, how long must a 3.0 g white gold broach be immersed to plate 3.0×10^{-5} g of rhodium? (Faraday's constant = 96,500 C/mol e^-)

A) 0.0009 s
B) 0.0098 s
C) 0.042 s
D) 0.56 s

7. A galvanic cell is constructed from two half-cells of platinum and iron. The half-reactions for these two elements are provided as follows:

$$Pt^{2+}(aq) + 2e^- \rightarrow Pt\ (s) \qquad E° = +1.20 \text{ V}$$
$$Fe^{3+}(aq) + 3e^- \rightarrow Fe\ (s) \qquad E° = -0.036 \text{ V}$$

Which of the following statements is true about the galvanic cell?

A) $E° = 1.164$ V, and Pt^{2+} is the reducing agent
B) $E° = 1.164$ V, and Fe^{3+} is the reducing agent.
C) $E° = 1.236$ V, and Pt^{2+} is the oxidizing agent.
D) $E° = 1.236$ V, and Fe^{3+} is the oxidizing agent.

8. An electrochemical cell is constructed using two inert electrodes in one chamber with an inert electrolyte. The binary compound ICl is dissolved in the electrolyte, current is applied, and I_2 and Cl_2 are produced. Which of the following statements is true?

A) Cl_2 was produced by reduction at the cathode.
B) I_2 was produced by oxidation at the cathode.
C) Cl_2 was produced by oxidation at the cathode.
D) I_2 was produced by reduction at the cathode.

CHAPTER 12 PRACTICE PASSAGE

A student performed an extensive experiment to determine the relative rates of corrosion of various metals with a variety of strong acids. The experimental procedure involved immersing three sets of ten 1.0-gram metal samples into three different acid baths, and then quantifying the reaction's spontaneity based upon the vigor of gas evolution. Reactions were designated as being either *violent* (X), *vigorous* (V), *moderate* (M), *sluggish* (S), or *nonspontaneous* (OO). The reactions were performed in a Styrofoam calorimeter. Gas evolution was monitored visually, and the heat evolved in the bath C reactions (data not given here) was measured with a calibrated thermometer. All reactions in bath C were allowed to go to completion.

Metal	Bath A	Bath B	Bath C
Magnesium	V	V	X
Lead	OO	OO	V
Iron	M	S	X
Aluminum	V	M	X
Copper	OO	OO	V
Silver	OO	OO	M
Zinc	V	V	X
Cobalt	M	M	X
Tin	M	M	V
Mercury	OO	OO	M

Table 1 Rates of gas evolution

Reagents:

Bath A contained hydrochloric acid (12 M)
Bath B contained sulfuric acid (18 M)
Bath C contained nitric acid (16 M)

Based upon his observations, the student constructed two linear rankings of the reduction potentials of the acids and the metals. The first ranking was based solely upon the qualitative rates of gas evolution as listed above, and the second ranking was based solely upon his quantitative Bath C heat data.

He found that his first table was in general agreement with previously published reductions tables, although pairs of metals with similar reduction potentials were in reversed order half of the time. Yet surprisingly, his second table had no correlation with any accepted work. It assigned Al and Mg with potentials far too high (negative 10 and 12 volts), and gave mercury, silver, and lead values much smaller than what they should have been.

1. Based upon his first reduction potential table, the student correctly listed the metal with the highest (most positive) reduction potential as:

A) silver.
B) copper.
C) magnesium.
D) lead.

2. Which of the following statements is inconsistent with the *student's* data?

A) The nitrate ion has a higher reduction potential than H^+.
B) The nitrate ion is a better oxidizing agent than H^+.
C) The sulfate ion is a better oxidizing agent than H^+.
D) H^+, Cl^- and SO_4^{2-} must all have lower reduction potentials than lead, silver, copper, and mercury.

3. Based on the compiled rankings from columns A and B, which of the following neutral metals would be the most stable in a concentrated aqueous solution of CoI_2?

A) Iron
B) Zinc
C) Tin
D) Lead

4. Not surprisingly, the student's thermodynamic data failed to produce the accepted reduction potential table because he made some fundamental mistakes in this portion of his experiment. Which one of the following did NOT contribute to the huge experimental error?

A) In measuring and contrasting the heats of reactions of several compounds with differing molecular weights, the student should have used equal moles of reactants, not equal masses.
B) The acids in the immersion baths should have been the same concentration.
C) For reactions in which gaseous products are generated, one should use a sealed calorimeter with an airtight lid.
D) The specific heats of each of the systems were not taken into account, and may have differed.

5. As noted in the passage, the data in columns A and B are similar, but different from the data in column C. Which of the following acids would most likely re-create the data found in column C?

A) HBr
B) H_3PO_4
C) HF
D) $HClO_4$

SOLUTIONS TO CHAPTER 12 FREESTANDING PRACTICE QUESTIONS

1. **B**   Increasing reagent quantity has no effect on voltage (Item I is incorrect, eliminating choices A and C), and placing batteries in parallel would leave the voltage unchanged (Item II is incorrect, eliminating choice D). Oxidation of zinc takes place at the anode, and sodium is a better reducing agent than zinc due to its lower ionization energy and tendency to give up an electron (Item III would result in an increase in voltage; the correct answer is choice B).

2. **D**   *Oxidant* and *reductant* are synonymous with *oxidizing agent* and *reducing agent*, respectively. Choices A and B are saying the same thing, so both can be eliminated. To compare the relative strengths of the ions as oxidizing agents, reverse the half reaction for Fe so that it reads as a reduction:

$$Pb^{2+} + 2e^- \rightarrow Pb(s) \quad E° = -0.13 \text{ V}$$

$$Fe^{2+} + 2e^- \rightarrow Fe(s) \quad E° = -0.45 \text{ V}$$

Note that the sign of $E°$ is reversed in this process. Pb^{2+} has a more positive reduction potential than Fe^{2+}, making it the better oxidant.

3. **D**   This question is asking about two factors (a two by two question): $\Delta G°$ and $E°$, which are related by $\Delta G° = -nFE°$. For any spontaneous reaction, the change in Gibbs free energy ($\Delta G°$) is always less than 0 (eliminate choices A and C). As shown in the equation above, the standard reduction potential ($E°$) must be positive when $\Delta G°$ is negative, so eliminate choice B.

4. **B**   A large, positive reduction potential indicates a strong tendency to be reduced, and hence ability to act as an oxidizing agent. The question states that high-valent metals act as strong oxidizing agents. Examining the oxidation states of the metals in question, we see that Fe = +3, Os = +8, Zn = +2, and W = 0. Therefore, since Os bears the largest positive oxidation state, we know that it is the strongest oxidizing agent.

5. **C**   The anode is always the site of oxidation and the cathode is always the site of reduction; therefore, electrons always flow from the anode (oxidation) to the cathode (reduction) regardless of the kind of cell (choices A and D are wrong). In a galvanic cell, a spontaneous reaction liberates electrons and they flow freely to the positive electrode, which in this case would be the cathode. However, in an electrolytic cell the current is forcing the electrons to flow where they don't want to go: the negative electrode. In this case the cathode would be the negative electrode (choice B is wrong).

6. **C** Since current (I) = charge(Q)/time(t) we can set up and solve the following equation keeping in mind that the rhodium reduction in question is $Rh^{3+} + 3e^- \rightarrow Rh(s)$.

$$t = \frac{Q}{I} = \frac{(3 \times 10^{-5}\,g)\left(\dfrac{1\,mol\,Rh}{102.9\,g}\right)\left(\dfrac{3\,mol\,e^-}{1\,mol\,Rh}\right)\left(\dfrac{9.65 \times 10^4\,C}{1\,mol\,e^-}\right)}{2.0\,A}$$

$$t \approx \frac{(3 \times 10^{-5}\,g)\left(\dfrac{1\,mol\,Rh}{100\,g}\right)\left(\dfrac{3\,mol\,e^-}{1\,mol\,Rh}\right)\left(\dfrac{1.0 \times 10^5\,C}{1\,mol\,e^-}\right)}{2.0\,A} \approx \frac{9 \times 10^{-2}\,C}{2.0\,A} \approx 0.045\,s$$

7. **C** The half-reaction with the *less positive* reduction potential (in this case, $Fe^{3+}(aq) + 3e^- \rightarrow$ Fe(s)) should be reversed in order to combine the half-reactions to obtain an $E^o > 0$ and create a galvanic cell. When the Fe half-reaction is reversed, the sign of the potential must be reversed. Combining the two half-reactions then gives: $3\,Pt^{2+}(aq) + 2\,Fe(s) \rightarrow 2\,Fe^{3+}(aq) + 3\,Pt(s)$ with an $E^o = 1.236$ V (eliminate choices A and B). Since Fe^{3+} is the product of the reaction, it cannot be the oxidizing agent (eliminate choice D). However, Pt^{2+} is reduced (it gains electrons from the Fe that is oxidized), so it is therefore the oxidizing agent.

8. **D** In the compound ICl, I has an +1 oxidation state, and Cl has a –1 oxidation state owing to the greater electronegativity of Cl. Therefore, production of Cl_2 must be an oxidation, and production of I_2 must be a reduction eliminating choices A and B. Moreover, reduction always takes place at the cathode, eliminating choice C.

SOLUTIONS TO CHAPTER 12 PRACTICE PASSAGE

1. **A** A metal with a high reduction potential will not be easily oxidized by the H^+ in the acid. The student's data indicated that choices B, C, and D were more reactive with acids than choice A.

2. **C** Of all the strong acids in the passage, only nitric acid and sulfuric acid have conjugate bases with positive reduction potentials. Choices A and B are correct, nitric acid is more corrosive than sulfuric and hydrochloric acid because the nitrate ion has a higher reduction potential (is a better oxidizing agent) than H^+. This is supported by data in the table. Choice D is also correct because the ions present in Bath A and Bath B were unable (had a lower reduction potential) to oxidize lead, silver, copper, and mercury—the student observed no reaction. If choice C is correct, sulfuric acid should be more corrosive than HCl, but this was not observed in the data set.

3. **D** The table indicates a moderate reaction when Co was added to either hydrochloric or sulfuric acid. Metals that react more readily than Co might be expected to have a greater preference for their oxidized state than Co does, which means that Co^{2+} likely oxidizes Zn, (eliminate choice B). The qualitative nature of the ranking does not indicate whether tin, cobalt, or iron have the highest reduction potential, but it does indicate that lead was inert in the acidic solutions, meaning it would be the most stable toward a concentrated Co^{2+} solution. This makes choice D the best answer.

4. **B** Choices A, C, and D would be serious errors. Since the metal samples were the limiting reagent, not the acids themselves, the concentration of the acids is irrelevant.

5. **D** HCl, H_2SO_4 and HNO_3 are all strong acids, and may undergo reduction through their H^+ entity resulting in the formation of H_2. However, the fact that the three columns are not the same indicates another mechanism of reduction. In this case, the highly oxidized nitrogen in the NO_3^- anion (formally N^{+5}) is capable of extracting electrons and forming nitrogen oxides with lower oxidation states. The most similar acid listed in this regard is $HClO_4$, which contains a highly oxidized formal Cl^{+7}. The remaining three acids may be expected, to one degree or another, to show reduction to H_2 in the presence of reducing equivalents, but none of these have such highly unstable electronegative elements in highly positive oxidation states. The phosphorous atom in H_3PO_4 is in a +5 state, but is much more like the S^{+6} atom in the stable SO_4^{2-} (column B) than the N^{+5} in NO_3^-.

Glossary

absolute zero
The temperature (–273.15°C or 0 K) at which the volume and pressure of an ideal gas extrapolate to zero according to the ideal gas law. [**Section 6.4**]

acid
See *Arrhenius acid*, *Brønsted-Lowry acid*, and *Lewis acid*. [**Section 11.1**]

acid-base indicator
A weak acid and conjugate base pair, such as litmus or phenolphthalein, that changes color with changes in solution pH. [**Section 11.1**]

acid-dissociation constant (K_a)
A measure of the extent of dissociation of an acid, HA. K_a is defined as $K_a = [H_3O^+][A^-]/[HA]$. [**Section 11.3**]

activation energy, E_a
The energy required by the reactants in a chemical reaction to reach a transition state from which the products of the reaction can form. [**Section 6.6**]

alkali metal
One of the metal elements in Group I (Li, Na, K, Rb, Cs, and Fr). [**Section 4.7**]

alkaline earth metal
One of the metal elements in Group II (Be, Mg, Ca, Sr, Ba, and Ra). [**Section 4.7**]

allotropes
Forms of a pure element with different structures and therefore different chemical and physical properties, such as O_2 and O_3 or carbon$_{(diamond)}$ and carbon$_{(graphite)}$. [**Section 6.6**]

alloy
A blend of two or more metallic elements. Bronze, for example, is an alloy of copper and tin. [**Section 10.4**]

alpha (α) particle
A positively charged particle consisting of two protons and two neutrons emitted during alpha decay. An alpha particle is identical to a helium-4 nucleus. [**Section 4.4**]

amphoteric
An ion or molecule, such as H_2O or HCO_3^-, that can act as either a Brønsted-Lowry acid or base. [**Section 11.3**]

anhydrous
A substance that is devoid of water. Used, for example, to differentiate between liquid (anhydrous) ammonia at temperatures below its boiling point (–33°C) and solutions of ammonia dissolved in water.

anion
A negatively charged ion, such as F⁻. [**Section 4.3**]

anode
The site of oxidation in a galvanic or electrolytic cell. Also, the electrode towards which anions flow through a salt bridge. [**Section 12.2**]

aqueous
Solutions of substances where water is the primary solvent. [**Section 10.4**]

Arrhenius acid
A compound that dissociates when it dissolves in water to give the H⁺ ion. [**Section 11.1**]

Arrhenius base
A compound that dissociates when it dissolves in water to give the OH⁻ ion. [**Section 11.1**]

Arrhenius equation
The equation for the rate constant (k) of a chemical reaction, in terms of the temperature (T), activation energy (E_a), and collision frequency/steric orientation factor (A): $k = Ae^{-E_a/RT}$. [**Section 9.4**]

atomic mass unit (amu, u)
The unit of mass most convenient for individual subatomic particles, atoms, and molecules. [**Section 3.6**]

atomic number (Z)
The number of protons in the nucleus of an atom. [**Section 4.1**]

atomic orbital
A region in space where electrons of an atom are most probably found. [**Section 5.2**]

atomic radius
The size of an atom equal to the volume of space carved out by the outermost (valence) electrons. [**Section 4.8**]

atomic weight
The weighted average of the atomic masses of the different isotopes of an element. A single ^{12}C atom, for example, has a mass of 12 amu, but naturally occurring carbon also contains 1.1% ^{13}C. The atomic weight of carbon is therefore 12.011 amu. [**Section 3.6**]

Aufbau principle
The principle that atomic orbitals are filled one at a time, starting with the orbital that has the lowest energy and then filling upwards. [**Section 4.6**]

Avogadro's number
The number of items that make up one mole, approximately 6.02×10^{23}. [**Section 3.7**]

Avogadro's hypothesis
The hypothesis that equal volumes of different gases at the same temperature and pressure contain the same number of particles. [**Section 8.2**]

base
See *Arrhenius base, Brønsted-Lowry base,* and *Lewis base.* [**Section 11.1**]

base-dissociation constant (K_b)
A measure of the extent of dissociation of a base, B: $K_b = [HB^+][OH^-]/[B]$. [**Section 11.3**]

battery
A set of electrochemical cells connected in series or parallel. [**Section 12.6**]

beta (β) decay
A nuclear reaction in which an electron (e^-) or positron (β^+) is absorbed by or emitted from the nucleus of an atom. [**Section 4.4**]

beta (β) particle
An electron or a positron. [**Section 4.4**]

bimolecular
A step in a chemical reaction in which two molecules collide to form products. [**Section 9.4**]

Bohr model
A model of the distribution of electrons in an atom based on the assumption that the electron in a hydrogen atom is in one of a limited number of circular orbits. [**Section 4.5**]

Bohr atom
An atom or ion that has just one electron such as H, He^+, Li^{2+}, etc. [**Section 4.5**]

boiling point
The temperature at which the vapor pressure of a liquid is equal to the external or atmospheric pressure. [**Section 5.8**]

bond-dissociation energy/enthalpy
The energy needed to homolytically break an X—Y bond to give X and Y atoms in the gas phase. [**Section 5.2**]

bonding electrons
A pair of electrons, always the outermost (valence) electrons, used to form a covalent bond between adjacent atoms. [**Section 5.1**]

Boyle's law
A statement of the relationship between the pressure and volume of a constant amount of gas at constant temperatures: $P \propto 1/V$. [**Section 8.2**]

Brønsted-Lowry acid
Any molecule or ion that can donate an H^+ (proton) to a base. [**Section 11.1**]

Brønsted-Lowry base
Any molecule or ion that can accept an H^+ (proton) from an acid. [Section 11.1]

buffer
A mixture of a weak acid (HA) and its conjugate base (A^-), which should be present in roughly equal amounts. Buffers resist a change in the pH of a solution according to Le Châtelier's principle when small amounts of acid or base are added. [Section 11.8]

buffer capacity
The amount of acid or base a buffer solution can absorb without significant changes in pH. [Section 11.8]

calorie
The heat needed to raise the temperature of 1 gram of water by 1°C. [Section 7.2]

calorimeter
An insulated apparatus used to measure the heat absorbed/released in a chemical reaction.

catalyst
A substance that increases the rate of a chemical reaction without being consumed in the reaction. [Section 3.13]
A substance that lowers the activation energy for a chemical reaction by providing an alternate pathway for the reaction. [Section 9.3]

cathode
The site of reduction in a galvanic or electrolytic cell. Also, the electrode in an electrochemical cell towards which cations flow through a salt bridge. [Section 12.2]

cation
A positively charged ion, such as Na^+. [Section 4.3]

cell potential
A measure of the driving force behind an electrochemical reaction, reported in volts. [Section 12.3]

Charles's law
A statement of the relationship between the temperature and volume of a constant amount of gas at constant pressure: $V \propto T$. [Section 8.3]

collision theory model
A model used to explain the rates of chemical reactions, which assumes that molecules must collide in order to react. [Section 9.2]

common-ion effect
The decrease in the solubility of a salt that occurs when the salt is dissolved in a solution that contains another source of one of its ions. Just another form of Le Châtelier's principle. [Section 10.6]

complex ion
An ion in which a ligand is bound to a metal via a coordinate covalent bond. An ion formed when a Lewis acid such as the Co^{2+} ion reacts with a Lewis base such as NH_3 to form an acid-base complex such as the $Co(NH_3)_4^{2+}$ ion. [Section 10.7]

compound
A substance with a constant composition that contains two or more elements.

concentration
A measure of the ratio of the amount of solute in a solution to the amount of either solvent or solution. Frequently expressed as molarity (units of moles of solute per liter of solution). [Section 3.9]

concentration cell
A type of electrochemical cell that has identical reactants in each half reaction, but at different concentrations, thus driving a weak electrical current. [Section 12.4]

conjugate acid-base pair
Two substances related by the gain or loss of a proton. An acid (such as HBr) and its conjugate base (Br^-), or a base (such as NH_3) and its conjugate acid (NH_4^+) are examples of conjugate acid-base pairs. [Section 11.3]

coordinate covalent bond
A covalent bond formed as a result of a Lewis acid-base reaction, most often formed between a metal atom and a nonmetal atom. [**Section 5.3**]

coordination compound
A compound in which one or more ligands are coordinated to a metal atom. [**Section 5.3**]

corrosion
A process in which a metal is destroyed by a chemical reaction. When the metal is iron, the process is called rusting.

covalent bond
A bond between two atoms formed by the sharing of at least one pair of electrons. [**Section 5.3**]

covalent compound
A compound, such as water (H_2O), composed of neutral molecules in which the atoms are held together by covalent bonds. [**Section 5.3**]

critical point
The temperature and pressure at which two phases of a substance that are in equilibrium (usually the gas and liquid phases) become identical and form a single phase. [**Section 7.4**]

crystal
A three-dimensional solid formed by regular repetition of the packing of atoms, ions, or molecules. [**Section 5.8**]

Dalton's law of partial pressures
A statement of the relationship between the total pressure of a mixture of gases and the partial pressures of the individual components: $P_{total} = p_1 + p_2 + p_3 + \ldots$. [**Section 8.4**]

daughter nucleus
The product nucleus after a nuclear reaction. [**Section 4.4**]

density
The mass of a sample divided by its volume. [**Section 3.2**]

deposition
A process in which a gas goes directly to the solid state without passing through an intermediate liquid state. [**Section 7.1**]

diamagnetic
A substance in which the electrons are all paired. [**Section 4.6**]

dilution
The process by which more solvent is added to decrease the concentration of a solution.

dimer
A compound (such as B_2H_6) produced by combining two smaller identical molecules (such as BH_3).

dipole
Anything with two equal but opposite electrical charges, such as the positive and negative ends of a polar bond or molecule. [**Section 5.6**]

diprotic acid
An acid, such as H_2SO_4, that can lose two H^+.

diprotic base
A base, such as the O^{2-} ion, that can accept two H^+.

dissolution
The process in which a bulk solid or liquid breaks up into individual molecules or ions and diffuses throughout a solvent. [**Section 10.4**]

ductile
Capable of being drawn into thin sheets or wires without breaking; a property of metals. [**Section 5.8**]

effusion
The process by which a gas escapes through a pinhole into a region of lower pressure. [**Section 8.5**]

elastic collision
A collision in which no kinetic energy is lost. [**Section 8.1**]

electrolyte

A substance that increases the electrical conductivity of water by dissociating into ions. [Section 10.1]

electrolysis

A process in which an electric current is used to drive a nonspontaneous chemical reaction. [Section 12.6]

electrolytic cell

A nonspontaneous electric cell in which electrolysis is done. [Section 12.6]

electron

A subatomic particle with a mass of only about 0.0005 amu and a charge of −1 that surrounds the nucleus of an atom. [Section 4.1]

electron affinity

The energy given off when a neutral atom in the gas phase picks up an electron to form a negatively charged ion. [Section 4.8]

electron capture

A type of beta decay where the nucleus of an atom captures an electron and converts a nuclear proton into a neutron. [Section 4.4]

electron configuration

The arrangement of electrons in atomic orbitals; for example, $1s^2 2s^2 2p^3$. [Section 4.6]

electronegativity

The tendency of an atom to draw or polarize bonding electrons toward itself. [Section 4.8]

element

A substance that cannot be decomposed into a simpler substance by a chemical reaction. A substance composed of only one kind of atom. [Section 3.6]

empirical formula

The formula for a compound in which the number of atoms of each element in the compound are represented by the lowest whole number ratio. [Section 3.4]

endergonic

A process that leads to an increase in the free energy of a system and is therefore not spontaneous: ΔG_{rxn} is positive. [Section 6.6]

endothermic

A chemical reaction that absorbs heat from the surroundings: ΔH_{rxn} is positive. [Section 6.2]

endpoint

The point at which the indicator of an acid-base titration changes color. [Section 12.5]

enthalpy (H)

The total potential energy in a substance due to intermolecular forces and covalent bonds. [Section 6.2]

enthalpy of reaction (ΔH_{rxn})

The change in the enthalpy that occurs during a chemical reaction. The difference between the sum of the enthalpies of the products and the reactants. [Section 6.2]

entropy (S)

A measure of the disorder in a system. Increasing disorder yields a positive ΔS. [Section 6.4]

equilibrium (dynamic)

The point at which there is no longer a change in the concentrations of the reactants and the products of a chemical reaction. The point at which the rates of the forward and reverse reactions are equal: $\Delta G_{rxn} = 0$. [Section 10.4]

equilibrium constant (K_{eq})

The product of the concentrations (or partial pressures) of the products of a reaction at equilibrium divided by the product of the concentrations (or partial pressures) of the reactants. [Section 10.1]

equilibrium expression

The expression used to calculate the equilibrium constant for a reaction that takes the form [products]/[reactants]. [Section 10.1]

equivalence point
The point in an acid-base titration at which the number of moles of H_3O^+ in solution equals the number of moles of OH^- in solution. [**Section 11.10**]

excited state configuration
One of an infinite number of electron configurations of an energized atom where at least one electron occupies an orbital of higher energy than that dictated by Hund's rule and/or the Aufbau principle. [**Section 4.5**]

exergonic
A process that leads to a decrease in the free energy of the system and is therefore spontaneous: ΔG_{rxn} is negative. [**Section 6.6**]

exothermic
A chemical reaction that releases energy to the surroundings: ΔH_{rxn} is negative. [**Section 6.2**]

family
A vertical column of elements in the periodic table, such as the elements Li, Na, K, etc. [**Section 4.6**]

Faraday's law of electrolysis
A statement of the relationship between the amount of electric current that passes through an electrolytic cell and the amount of product formed during electrolysis. The amount of chemical change is proportional to the amount of electric current that flows through the cell. [**Section 12.7**]

first ionization energy
The energy needed to remove the valence electron from a neutral atom in the gas phase. [**Section 4.8**]

first law of thermodynamics
The total energy in the universe is conserved: energy is neither created nor destroyed, but may change from one form to another. [**Section 6.1**]

first-order reaction
A reaction in which the rate is proportional to the concentration of a single reactant raised to the first power: rate = $k[A]$. [**Section 9.4**]

formal charge
The theoretical charge on an atom in a molecule, calculated by $V - \frac{1}{2}B - L$, where V is the number of valence electrons, B is the number of bonding electrons, and L is the number of lone-pair electrons. [**Section 5.1**]

free energy, Gibbs (G)
The energy associated with a chemical reaction that can be used to do work. The change in free energy of a system is calculated by the formula $\Delta G = \Delta H - T\Delta S$, where G is the free energy, H is enthalpy, T is temperature (in kelvins), and S is entropy. [**Section 6.5**]

free radical
An atom or molecule that contains an unpaired electron. [**Section 5.2**]

freezing point
The temperature at which the solid and liquid phases of a substance are in equilibrium. [**Section 7.1**]

fusion
The melting of a solid to form a liquid. [**Section 7.1**]

galvanic cell
An electrochemical cell that uses a spontaneous chemical reaction to do work. Synonymous with *voltaic cell*. [**Section 12.2**]

gamma ray (γ)
A high energy, short wavelength form of electromagnetic radiation emitted by the nucleus of an atom that carries off some of the energy generated in a nuclear reaction. [**Section 4.4**]

Gibbs free energy
See *free energy*. [**Section 6.5**]

Graham's law
The relationship between the rate at which a gas diffuses or effuses and its molecular weight: rate $\propto 1/(MW)^{1/2}$. [Section 8.5]

ground state configuration
The most stable arrangement of electrons in an atom that satisfies Hund's rule and the Aufbau principle. [Section 4.5]

group
A vertical column, or family, of elements in the periodic table. [Section 4.7]

half-life
The time required for the amount of a decaying substance to decrease to half its initial value. [Section 4.4]

halogen
Elements of Group VII: F, Cl, Br, I, and At. [Section 4.7]

heat (q)
Thermal energy in transit from a hotter system to a colder one. [Section 6.1]

heat of fusion
The heat that must be absorbed to melt a unit quantity of a solid. [Section 7.2]

heat of reaction
The change in the enthalpy of the system that occurs when a reaction is run at constant pressure. Synonymous with *enthalpy of reaction*, ΔH_{rxn}. [Section 6.2]

heat of vaporization
The heat that must be absorbed to boil a unit quantity of a liquid. [Section 7.2]

heat capacity
The amount of heat required to raise the temperature of a given amount of a substance by one degree. Not to be confused with *specific heat*. Heat capacity is typically the product of mass and specific heat. [Section 7.3]

Hess's law
The heat given off or absorbed in a chemical reaction does not depend on whether the reaction occurs in a single step or in many steps. [Section 6.3]

homonuclear diatomic molecule
A molecule, such as O_2 or F_2, that contains two atoms of the same element.

Hund's rule
Rule for placing electrons in equal-energy orbitals, which states that electrons are added with parallel spins until each of the orbitals has one electron, before a second electron is placed in a given orbital. [Section 4.6]

hybrid orbitals
Orbitals formed by mixing two or more atomic orbitals. [Section 5.5]

hybridization
A process in which things are mixed. A resonance hybrid is a mixture, or average, of two or more Lewis structures. Hybrid orbitals are formed by mixing two or more atomic orbitals. [Section 5.5]

hydride
The species H^-. [Section 5.4]

hydrogen bonding
A strong dipole-dipole interaction that occurs between a hydrogen atom covalently bonded to an F, O, or N that electrostatically interacts with a lone pair of electrons on another F, O, or N atom. [Section 5.7]

hydrophilic
"Water loving"; attracted or compatible with water (for example, ions that are soluble in water).

hydrophobic
"Water fearing"; repelled by or incompatible with water (for example, lipids that are insoluble in water).

ideal gas
A gas that obeys all the postulates of the kinetic-molecule theory and has properties that can be predicted by the ideal gas law. [Section 8.1]

ideal gas law
The relationship between the pressure, volume, temperature, and amount of an ideal gas: $PV = nRT$. [Section 8.2]

immiscible
Liquids, such as oil and water, that do not dissolve in one another.

indicator
See *acid-base indicator*. [Section 11.9]

induced dipole
A short-lived separation of charge, or dipole, of a nonpolar atom or molecule caused by the electrostatic influence of a nearby polar atom or ion. [Section 5.7]

inert
Unreactive. Used to describe compounds that do not undergo chemical reactions. [Section 4.7]

insoluble
Used to describe a substance that does not noticeably dissolve in a solvent. [Section 10.4]

intermolecular forces
Attractive electrostatic forces, the strength of which determine a compound's phase, vapor pressure, melting point, boiling point, solubility, and viscosity. From strongest to weakest, the main categories of intermolecular forces are: *ionic*, *dipole-dipole* (with H-bonds the strongest), and *London dispersion forces*. [Section 5.7]

intramolecular bonds
Synonym for covalent bonds. There are three primary types: normal covalent bonds, metallic covalent bonds, and coordinate covalent bonds. [Section 7.1]

ion product (Q_{sp})
The product of the concentrations of the ions in a solution at any moment. [Section 10.5]

ion-product constant of water (K_w)
The product of the equilibrium concentration of the H_3O^+ and OH^- ions in an aqueous solution at $25°C$: $K_w = 1.0 \times 10^{-14}$. [Section 11.4]

ionic bond
Misappropriation of the term *bond*. Simply the strong electrostatic attraction between two oppositely charged ions; there is no electron sharing. [Section 5.3]

ionic compound
A compound made up of ions (synonymous with *salt*). [Section 3.6]

ionizability factor (i)
The number of individual particles formed when an individual solute dissolves. Synonymous with *van't Hoff factor*. [Section 10.4]

ionization
A process in which an ion is created from a neutral atom or molecule by adding or removing one or more electrons. [Section 4.8]

ionization energy
See *first ionization energy*. [Section 4.8]

isoelectronic
Atoms or ions that have the same number of electrons and therefore the same electron configuration, such as O^{2-}, F^-, Ne, and Na^+. [Section 4.6]

isotopes
Nuclides of the same element, but with differing numbers of neutrons, such as ^{12}C, ^{13}C, and ^{14}C. Isotopes have nearly identical chemical properties. [Section 4.2]

joule
A unit of measurement for both heat and work in the SI system. 1 J = 4.184 cal. [Section 3.1]

kinetic energy
The energy associated with motion. The kinetic energy of an object is equal to one-half the product of its mass and the square of its speed: $KE = \frac{1}{2}mv^2$. [Section 5.7]

kinetic-molecular theory
The theory that states heat is associated with the thermal motion of particles, taking into account the important assumptions that individual gas molecules take up no volume and collisions between gas molecules are perfectly elastic. [Section 8.1]

Le Châtelier's principle
A principle that describes the effect of changes in the temperature, pressure, or concentration of one of the reactants or products of a reaction at equilibrium. It states that when a system at equilibrium is subjected to a stress, it will shift in the direction that minimizes the effect of this stress. [Section 10.3]

Lewis acid
An atom or molecule that accepts a pair of electrons to form a new coordinate covalent bond. Almost always a metal atom, positively charged ion, or both. [Section 5.3]

Lewis base
An atom or molecule that donates a pair of electrons to form a new coordinate covalent bond. Almost always a nonmetal with a pair of nonbonding electrons. Synonymous with *ligand* and *chelator*. [Section 5.3]

ligand
See *Lewis base*. [Section 5.3]

limiting reagent
The reactant in a chemical reaction that is exhausted first, thus limiting the amount of product that can be formed. [Section 3.12]

London dispersion forces
Intermolecular forces that arise from interactions between an instantaneous dipole/induced dipole pair. Typically, these are the weakest of all intermolecular forces. However LDFs are additive, and nonpolar molecules with large, flat surface areas can experience moderate LDFs. [Section 5.7]

malleable
Something that can be hammered, pounded, or pressed into different shapes without breaking (a common property of metals). [Section 5.8]

mass number (A)
The total number of protons and neutrons in the nucleus of an atom. [Section 4.1]

melting point
The temperature at which the solid and liquid phases of a substance are in equilibrium at a particular external pressure. [Section 5.7]

metal
An element that is solid, has a metallic luster, is malleable and ductile, and conducts both heat and electricity. [Section 3.10]

metalloid
An element with properties that fall between the extremes of metals and nonmetals. [Section 4.7]

mixture
A substance that contains two or more elements or compounds that retain their chemical identities and can be separated by a physical process. For example, the mixture of N_2 and O_2 in the atmosphere. [Section 3.9]

molarity (M)
The number of moles of a solute in a solution divided by the volume of the solution in liters. [Section 3.1]

mole
6.02×10^{23} of anything. [Section 3.7]

mole fraction (X)
The fraction of the total number of moles in a mixture due to one component of the mixture. The mole fraction of a solute, for example, is the number of moles of solute divided by the total number of moles of solute plus solvent. [Section 3.9]

mole ratio
The ratio of the moles of one reactant or product to the moles of another reactant or product in the balanced equation for a chemical reaction.

molecular formula
The formula representing the number and type of constituent atoms in a compound. [Section 3.3]

molecular geometry
The arrangement of atoms surrounding a central atom of a small molecule. Molecular geometry (or the shape of a molecule) and orbital geometry are identical only when the central atom possesses no lone pairs of electrons. [Section 5.4]

molecular weight
The weight of the molecular formula, calculated from a table of atomic weights. Note that atomic weights are a weighted average of masses of isotopes as they occur in nature. [Section 5.7]

molecule
The smallest particle that has any of the chemical or physical properties of a compound. [Section 3.3]

monoprotic acid (HA)
An acid, such as HF or HOCl, that can lose only one H^+.

negative electrode
The electrode in an electrochemical cell that carries a negative charge. In a galvanic cell, it is the anode; in an electrolytic cell, it is the cathode.

Nernst equation
Used to calculate or track the voltage of an electrochemical cell under *nonstandard* conditions: $E = E° - (0.06/n) \log Q$. [Section 12.4]

network solid
A solid, such as diamond, in which every atom is covalently bonded to its nearest neighbors to form an extended array of atoms rather than individual molecules. [Section 5.8]

neutron
A subatomic particle with a mass of about 1 amu and no charge. [Section 4.1]

noble gases
The elements in the last column of the periodic table that are chemically unreactive. [Section 4.6]

nonbonding electrons
Electrons in the valence shell of an atom that are not used to form covalent bonds. [Section 5.1]

nonmetal
An element that lacks the properties generally associated with metals. These elements are found in the upper right of the periodic table. [Section 4.7]

nonpolar
Used to describe a compound that has a homogenous electron distribution and thus does not carry a permanent dipole moment. [Section 5.3]

nonspontaneous
A reaction in which the products are not favored, implying that the reverse reaction would be favored: ΔG_{rxn} is positive (and E_{cell} is negative). [Section 2.6]

nucleon
Generic term for a proton or neutron. [Section 4.1]

nuclide

The generic term for any particular isotope of an element, such as the ^{13}C nuclide.

octet rule

The tendency of main-group elements to react in order to possess eight valence-shell electrons in their compounds.

orbital geometry

The arrangement of electron clouds surrounding a central atom of a small molecule. Orbital geometry is a consequence of hybridization. Not to be confused with *shape*, or *molecular geometry*. [Section 5.4]

orbitals

Regions in space where electrons have a high probability of existing. [Section 4.5]

order

Used to describe the relationship between the rate of a step in a chemical reaction and the concentration of one of the reactants consumed in that step. Essentially just the value of the exponent found in a reactant term in the rate law. [Section 9.4]

oxidation

A process in which an atom, ion, or molecule loses one or more electrons. [Section 3.14]

oxidation number

Synonymous with *oxidation state*. It is the hypothetical charge that would be present on each atom if a molecule was shattered into its individual constituent atoms with bonding electrons ending up with the atom of the bond having the higher electronegativity. [Section 3.14]

oxidation-reduction reaction

A chemical reaction involving the exchange of electrons such that oxidation numbers of reactants change. [Section 12.1]

oxidizing agent / oxidant

An atom, ion, or molecule that undergoes reduction by gaining electrons, thereby oxidizing something else. [Section 4.7]

pH

A measure of acidity ranging from about -1.5 to 15.5 in aqueous media, defined as $-\log [H_3O^+]$. [Section 11.5]

pOH

The complement of pH, defined as $-\log [OH^-]$. [Section 11.5]

paramagnetic

A compound that contains one or more unpaired electrons and is attracted into a magnetic field. [Section 4.6]

parent nucleus

The initial nucleus prior to a nuclear reaction. [Section 4.4]

partial pressure

The fraction of the total pressure of a mixture of gases that is due to one component of the mixture. As molarity is the primary way of expressing the amount of solute in a solution, so too is partial pressure the primary way to report the quantity of a gas in a mixture of gases. [Section 8.4]

Pauli exclusion principle

The maximum number of electrons in any given orbital is two, and they must have the opposite spin. [Section 4.6]

period

A horizontal row in the periodic table. [Section 4.6]

polar covalent bond

A covalent bond between atoms with differing electronegativities such that electrons spend more time in the vicinity of one atom than the other.

polar
Used to describe a molecule that has a dipole moment because it consists of a positive pole and a negative pole. [**Section 5.3**]

polyatomic ion
An ion that contains more than one atom, such as CO_3^{2-} or SO_4^{2-}. [**Section 3.5**]

polyprotic acid
An acid, such as H_2SO_4 or H_3PO_4, that can lose more than one H^+. [**Section 11.3**]

polyprotic base
A base, such as the PO_4^{3-} ion, that can accept more than one H^+.

positive electrode
The electrode in an electrochemical cell that carries a positive charge. In a galvanic cell, it is the cathode; in an electrolytic cell, it is the anode.

positron (β^+)
The antiparticle of the electron. A positron has the same mass as an electron but is positively charged. Contact between an electron and positron results in instant annihilation and emission of two high energy gamma rays. [**Section 4.4**]

positron emission
A mode of beta decay where a positron is emitted as a consequence of the conversion of a nuclear proton to a neutron. [**Section 4.4**]

potential
A measure of the driving force behind an electrochemical reaction that is reported in units of volts. [**Section 12.3**]

precipitation
A process where dissolved ions combine to form a solid salt in solution. [**Section 10.4**]

precision
A measure of the extent to which individual measurements of the same phenomenon agree.

pressure
The force exerted perpendicular to a surface divided by the area of the surface. [**Section 5.7**]

proton
A subatomic particle that has a charge of +1 and a mass of about 1 amu. (Synonymous with H^+.) [**Section 4.1**]

quantized
A property or quality that appears only in certain discrete amounts, such as electric charge. [**Section 4.5**]

radioactivity
The spontaneous disintegration of an unstable nuclide by a first-order rate law. Synonymous with *nuclear decay*. [**Section 4.4**]

rate of reaction
The change in the concentration of a compound divided by the amount of time necessary for this change to occur: rate = $\Delta[X]/\Delta t$. [**Section 9.1**]

rate constant (k)
The proportionality constant in the equation that describes the relationship between the rate of a step in a chemical reaction and the product of the concentrations of the reactants consumed in that step. [**Section 9.4**]

rate law
An equation that describes how the rate of a chemical reaction depends on the concentrations of the reactants consumed in that reaction, along with the rate constant that takes into account temperature, activation energy, and collision frequency/steric effects. [**Section 9.4**]

rate-determining step
The slowest step in a chemical reaction. [**Section 9.1**]

reaction quotient (Q)
The quotient obtained when the concentrations (or partial pressures) of the products of a reaction are multiplied and the result is divided by the product of the concentrations (or partial pressures) of the reactants. Basically, putting nonequilibrium values into an equilibrium expression yields a reaction quotient instead of the equilibrium constant. [Section 10.2]

real gas
A gas that deviates from the behavior predicted by the ideal gas law. Real gases differ from the expected behavior of an ideal gas (e.g., lower V and P) for two reasons: (1) the forces of attraction between the particles in a gas are not zero and (2) the volume of the particles in a gas is not zero. [Section 8.3]

redox
An abbreviation for oxidation-reduction. [Section 12.1]

reducing agent / reductant
An atom, ion, or molecule that is oxidized by giving up electrons, thereby reducing something else. [Section 12.1]

reduction
A process in which an atom, ion, or molecule gains one or more electrons. [Section 12.1]

resonance structures
Two or more Lewis dot structures that differ only by the placement of electrons in the molecule. Taken together as an average (a resonance hybrid), they best approximate the electron distribution and types of bonds in the molecule better than any one structure can alone. [Section 5.1]

salt
Synonymous with *ionic compound*. [Section 5.8]

salt bridge
An ion-rich junction between the anodic and cathodic chambers of an electrochemical cell that prevents charge separation that would otherwise stop the cell from functioning. Anions always migrate toward the anode, and cations always migrate toward the cathode of any cell. [Section 12.2]

saturated solution
A solution that contains as much solute as possible. [Section 10.4]

second ionization energy
The energy needed to remove an electron from a +1 cation in the gas phase. [Section 4.8]

second law of thermodynamics
Processes that increase the entropy in the universe are spontaneous. [Section 6.4]

second-order reaction
A reaction in which rate is proportional to the concentration of a single reactant raised to the second power: rate = $k[A]^2$, or two reactants each raised to the first power: rate = $k[A][B]$.

shielding
The masking and weakening of the electrostatic attraction between the nucleus and outer electrons by inner electrons. [Section 4.8]

solubility
The ratio of the maximum amount of solute to the volume of solvent in which this solute can dissolve. Often expressed in units of grams of solute per 100 g of water, or in moles of solid per liter of solution. [Section 10.4]

solubility equilibria
Equilibria that exist in a saturated solution, in which additional solid dissolves at the same rate that particles of solution come together to precipitate more solid.

solubility product (K_{sp})
The product of the equilibrium concentrations of the ions in a saturated solution of a salt. [**Section 10.1**]

solute
The substance that dissolves in a solvent to form a solution. [**Section 10.4**]

solution
A homogeneous mixture of one or more solutes dissolved in a solvent. [**Section 10.4**]

solvent
The substance in which a solute dissolves. [**Section 10.4**]

specific heat
The amount of heat required to raise the temperature of 1 g of a substance by 1°C (or 1 K). (Do not confuse with *heat capacity*). [**Section 7.2**]

spontaneous reaction
A reaction in which the products are favored: ΔG_{rxn} is negative (and E_{cell} is positive). [**Section 6.5**]

standard cell potential
The potential, $E°_{cell}$, of a cell measured under standard-state conditions.

standard heat of formation ($\Delta H_f°$)
The change in the enthalpy that occurs during a chemical reaction that leads to the formation of one mole of a compound from its elements in their standard states at standard conditions. [**Section 6.3**]

standard state/condition
State in which T = 298 K (25°C), P = 1 atm, and all concentrations are 1 M. Not to be confused with STP. [**Section 6.3**]

standard temperature and pressure (STP)
State in which T = 273 K (0°C) and P = 1 atm. Generally used when referring to gases. Not to be confused with *standard state* or *standard conditions*. [**Section 6.3**]

state
1. One of the three states of matter: gas, liquid, or solid.

2. A set of physical properties that describe a system. [**Section 3.13**]

state function
A quantity whose value depends only on the state of the system and not its history; X is a state function, if and only if, the value of ΔX does not depend on the path used to go from the initial to the final state of the system. [**Section 6.3**]

stoichiometry
The study of the quantitative relationships between the reactants and the products of a balanced chemical reaction. [**Sections 3.10–3.12**]

strong acid
An acid that dissociates completely in water. [**Section 11.3**]

strong base
A base that dissociates completely in water. [**Section 11.3**]

sublimation
The process in which a solid goes directly to the gas phase without passing through an intermediate liquid state. [**Section 6.4**]

supercooled liquid
A substance that is a liquid even though its temperature is below its freezing point.

supercritical fluid
A substance that displays properties of both a liquid and a gas and exists under conditions of high temperature and pressure. If a substance is in this state—where the liquid and gas phases are no longer distinct—no amount of increased pressure can force the substance back into its liquid phase. [Section 7.4]

surface tension
The perpendicular force per unit length of liquid surface that acts to reduce the surface area of a liquid, resulting from intermolecular forces below the surface.

surroundings
In thermodynamics, the part of the universe not included in the system. [Section 6.1]

system
In thermodynamics, that small portion of the universe in which we are interested at the moment. [Section 6.1]

thermal conductor
A substance or object that readily conducts heat (metals, for example).

thermal insulator
An object, such as a blanket or a fur coat, that tends to slow down the rate at which heat is transferred from one object to another.

titrant
The strong acid or base reagent added to the unknown solution in a titration experiment. [Section 11.10]

titration
A technique used to determine the concentration and/or the chemical identity of a solute in a solution. [Section 11.10]

torr
A unit of pressure equal to the pressure exerted by a column of mercury 1 millimeter tall. By definition, 1 torr = 1 mm Hg. [Section 8.1]

transition metal
Metals in the block of elements that serve as a transition between the two columns on the left side of the table, where s orbitals are filled, and the six columns on the right, where p orbitals are filled. [Section 3.14]

triple point
The unique pressure and temperature at which the three phases of a substance (gas, liquid, and solid) can all coexist in equilibrium. [Section 7.4]

unimolecular
Describes a step in a reaction mechanism in which only one reactant molecule is present. [Section 9.4]

valence electrons
Electrons in the outermost or highest-energy level or shell of an atom. The electrons that are gained, shared, or lost in a chemical reaction. [Section 3.14]

van der Waals equation
An equation that accounts for deviations from ideal behavior in gaseous systems due to interactions between gas particles and particle volume. [Section 8.3]

van't Hoff factor (i)
See *ionizability factor*. [Section 10.4]

vapor pressure
The partial pressure of the gas molecules over the surface of a liquid that originate from the surface of a liquid. [Section 5.7]

voltaic cell
An electrochemical cell in which a spontaneous chemical reaction is used to create electricity. Synonymous with *galvanic cell*. [Section 12.2]

volatile
The physical characteristic of having a high vapor pressure at standard conditions. [Section 5.7]

VSEPR theory
A model in which the repulsion between pairs of
valence electrons is used to predict the shape of a
molecule. [**Section 5.4**]

weak acid
An acid that only partially dissociates in water.
[**Section 11.3**]

weak base
A base that only partially dissociates in water.
[**Section 11.3**]

zero-order reaction
A reaction in which rate is not proportional to the
concentration of any of the reactants.

MCAT G-Chem
Formula Sheet

Stoichiometry

Avogadro's number: $N_A = 6.02 \times 10^{23}$

$$\text{\# moles} = \frac{\text{mass in grams}}{\text{MW}}$$

$$\text{\% composition by mass of } X = \frac{\text{mass of X}}{\text{mass of molecule}} \times 100\%$$

$$\text{Mole fraction: } X_S = \frac{\text{moles of S}}{\text{total moles}}$$

$$\text{Molarity : } M = \frac{\text{moles of solute}}{\text{L of solution}}$$

Nuclear and Atomic Chemistry

N_A amu (u) = 1 gram

$$E_{\text{photon}} = hf = hc/\lambda$$

electron energy: $E_n = \dfrac{(-2.178 \times 10^{-18}\,\text{J})}{n^2}$ for any 1-electron (Bohr) atom

Z = # of protons = atomic number, N = # of neutrons

$A = Z + N$ = mass number

Decay	Description	ΔZ	ΔN	ΔA
α	eject $\alpha = {}^4_2\text{He}$	−2	−2	−4
β^-	$n \rightarrow p + e^-$	+1	−1	0
β^+	$p \rightarrow n + e^+$	−1	+1	0
EC	$p + e^- \rightarrow n$	−1	+1	0
γ	$X^* \rightarrow X + \gamma$	0	0	0

Bonding and Intermolecular Forces

formal charge: $FC = V - (\frac{1}{2}B + L)$

V = (# of valence e^-s)

B = (# of bonding e^-s)

L = (# of lone-pair e^-s)

VSEPR Theory

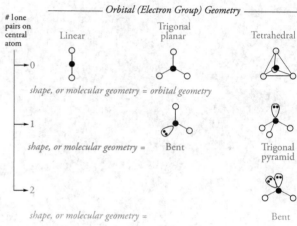

intermolecular forces (D=dipole, I=induced, i=instantaneous):

ion–ion > ion–D > H-bonds > D–D > D–ID > iD–ID (London dispersion)

Periodic Trends

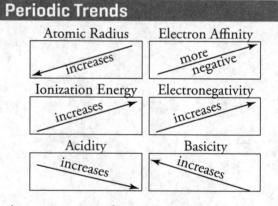

electronegativity of some common atoms:

F > O > (N ≈ Cl) > Br > (I ≈ S ≈ C) > H

Thermodynamics

T (in K) $= T_{°C} + 273$, 1 cal ≈ 4.2 J, $q =$ heat

$q = mc\Delta T = C\Delta T$ (if no phase changes)

$q = n\Delta H_{\text{phase change}}$ ($\Delta T = 0$ during phase change)

enthalpy change: $\Delta H =$ heat of rxn at const P

$\Delta H < 0 \Leftrightarrow$ exothermic, $\Delta H > 0 \Leftrightarrow$ endothermic

standard state: 1 M, 25°C, 1 atm

$\Delta H°_{\text{rxn}} = \sum n\Delta H°_{\text{f,products}} - \sum n\Delta H°_{\text{f,reactants}}$

Laws of Thermodynamics ($E =$ energy, $S =$ entropy):

1) E_{universe} is constant. $\Delta E_{\text{system}} = Q - W$.

2) Spontaneous rxn $\Rightarrow \Delta S_{\text{universe}} > 0$

3) $S = 0$ for pure crystal at $T = 0$ K

Gibbs Free Energy: $\Delta G = \Delta H - T\Delta S$ [const.T]

$\Delta G < 0 \Leftrightarrow$ forward reaction is spontaneous

$\Delta G = 0 \Leftrightarrow$ at equilibrium

$\Delta G > 0 \Leftrightarrow$ reverse reaction is spontaneous

$\Delta G° = -RT \ln K \approx -2.3RT \log K$

Gases

STP:

$T = 0$ °C $= 273$ K, $P = 1$ atm $= 760$ torr $= 760$ mmHg

Avogadro's Law: $V \propto n$

$$V_{\text{at STP}} = n(22.4 \text{ L})$$

Boyle's Law: $V \propto 1/P$ (at constant T)

Charles's Law: $V \propto T$ (at constant P)

Combined Gas Law: $P_1V_1/T_1 = P_2V_2/T_2$

Ideal Gas Law: $PV = nRT$

van der Waals: $\left(P + \dfrac{an^2}{V^2}\right)(V - nb) = nRT$

Dalton's law of partial pressures: $P_{\text{tot}} = \sum p_i$

Graham's law of effusion:

$$v_{2,rms} = v_{1,rms}\sqrt{\frac{m_1}{m_2}} \Rightarrow \frac{\text{rate of effusion of gas 2}}{\text{rate of effusion of gas 1}} = \sqrt{\frac{m_1}{m_2}}$$

Kinetics

Concentration rate =

$$-\frac{\Delta[\text{reactant}]}{\text{time}} \quad \text{or} \quad +\frac{\Delta[\text{product}]}{\text{time}}$$

Reaction rate =

$$-\frac{1}{\text{coeff}}\frac{\Delta[\text{reactant}]}{\text{time}} \quad \text{or} \quad +\frac{1}{\text{coeff}}\frac{\Delta[\text{product}]}{\text{time}}$$

Rate law for rate-determining step:

$$\text{rate} = k[\text{reactant}_1]^{\text{coeff}_1}\ldots$$

Arrhenius equation: $k = Ae^{-E_a/RT}$

Equilibrium

For generic balanced reaction

$aA + bB \rightleftharpoons cC + dD$,

equilibrium constant: $K_{\text{eq}} = \dfrac{[C]^c_{\text{at eq}}[D]^d_{\text{at eq}}}{[A]^a_{\text{at eq}}[B]^b_{\text{at eq}}}$ (excluding pure solids and liquids)

(gas rxns use partial pressures in K_p expression)

K_{eq} is a constant at a given temperature

$K_{\text{eq}} < 1 \Leftrightarrow$ equilibrium favors reactants

$K_{\text{eq}} > 1 \Leftrightarrow$ equilibrium favors products

Reaction quotient: $Q = \dfrac{[C]^c[D]^d}{[A]^a[B]^b}$

Le Châtelier's Principle

$Q < K_{\text{eq}} \Leftrightarrow$ rxn proceeds in a forward direction

$Q = K_{\text{eq}} \Leftrightarrow$ rxn at equilibrium

$Q > K_{\text{eq}} \Leftrightarrow$ rxn proceeds in a reverse direction

Acids and Bases

$pH = -\log[H^+] = -\log[H_3O^+]$

$pOH = -\log[OH^-]$

$K_w = [H^+][OH^-] = 1 \times 10^{-14}$ at 25 °C

$pH + pOH = 14$ at 25 °C

$K_a = \dfrac{[H^+][A^-]}{[HA]}$

$pK_a = -\log K_a$

$K_b = \dfrac{[OH^-][HB^+]}{[B]}$

$pK_b = -\log K_b$

$K_a K_b = K_w =$ ion-product constant for water

Henderson-Hasselbalch equations:

$$pH = pK_a + \log\dfrac{[\text{conjugate base}]}{[\text{weak acid}]}$$

$$= pK_a - \log\dfrac{[\text{weak acid}]}{[\text{conjugate base}]}$$

$$pOH = pK_b + \log\dfrac{[\text{conjugate acid}]}{[\text{weak base}]}$$

$$= pK_b - \log\dfrac{[\text{weak base}]}{[\text{conjugate acid}]}$$

acid-base neutralization:

$$a \times [A] \times V_A = b \times [B] \times V_B$$

Redox and Electrochemistry

Rules for determining oxidation state (OS):[*]

1) OS of pure element = 0

2) sum of OS's = 0 in neutral molecule

   sum of OS's = charge on ion

3) Group 1 metals: OS = +1

   Group 2 metals: OS = +2

4) OS of F = −1

5) OS of H = +1

6) OS of O = −2

7) OS of halogens = −1 of O family = −2

If one rule contradicts another, rule higher in list takes precedence.

$F =$ faraday $= 96{,}500$ C/mol e^-

$\Delta G = -nFE_{cell}$

$E_{cell} > 0 \Leftrightarrow$ spontaneous

$E_{cell} < 0 \Leftrightarrow$ reverse rxn is spontaneous

Nernst equation: $E = E° - \dfrac{0.06}{n}\log Q$

Faraday's Law of Electrolysis:

The amount of chemical charge is proportional to the amount of electricity that flows through the cell.

---

[*] These rules work 99 percent of the time.

MCAT Math for
General Chemistry

PREFACE

The MCAT is primarily a conceptual exam, with little actual mathematical computation. Any math that is on the MCAT is fundamental: just arithmetic, algebra, and trigonometry (and there is virtually no trigonometry in General Chemistry). There is absolutely no calculus. The purpose of this section of the book is to go over some math topics (as they pertain to General Chemistry) with which you may feel a little rusty[1].

This text is intended for reference and self-study. Therefore, there are lots of examples, all completely solved. Practice working through these examples and master the fundamentals!

Chapter 13
Arithmetic, Algebra, and Graphs

13.1 THE IMPORTANCE OF APPROXIMATION

Since you aren't allowed to use a calculator on the MCAT, you need to practice doing arithmetic calculations by hand again. Fortunately, the amount of calculation you'll have to do is small, and you'll also be able to approximate. For example, let's say you were faced with performing the following calculation:

$$
\begin{array}{r}
23.6 \\
\times\ 72.5 \\
\hline
1180 \\
472\ \ \\
1652\ \ \ \ \\
\hline
1711.00
\end{array}
$$

Your first inclination would be to reach for your calculator, but...you don't have one available. Now what? Realize that on the Chemical and Physical Foundations of Biological Systems section of the MCAT, you have roughly a minute and twenty-five seconds per question, so there simply cannot be questions requiring lengthy, complicated computation. Instead, we'll figure out a reasonably accurate (and fast) approximation of the value of the expression above:

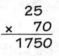

$$
\begin{array}{r}
25 \\
\times\ 70 \\
\hline
1750
\end{array}
$$

So, if the answer to an MCAT question was the value of the expression above, and the four answer choices were, say, 1324, 1617, 1711, and 1856, we'd know right away that the answer is 1711. The choices are far enough apart that even with our approximations, we were still able to tell which choice was the correct one. Just as importantly, we didn't waste time trying to be more precise; it was unnecessary, and it would have decreased the amount of time we had to spend on other questions.

If you find yourself writing out lengthy calculations on your scratch paper when you're working through MCAT questions that contain some mathematical calculation, it's important that you recognize that you're not using your time efficiently. Say to yourself, "I'm wasting valuable time trying to get a precise answer, when I don't need to be precise."

Try this one: What's 1583 divided by 32.1? (You have five seconds. Go.)

For the previous practice exercise, you should have written (or done in your head): $\dfrac{1500}{30} = 50$

13.2 SCIENTIFIC NOTATION, EXPONENTS, AND RADICALS

It's well known that very large or very small numbers can be handled more easily when they're written in **scientific notation**, that is, in the form $\pm\, m \times 10^n$, where $1 \le m < 10$ and n is an integer. For example:

$$602{,}000{,}000{,}000{,}000{,}000{,}000{,}000 = 6.02 \times 10^{23}$$
$$-35{,}000{,}000{,}000 = -3.5 \times 10^{10}$$
$$0.000000004 = 4 \times 10^{-9}$$

Quantities like these come up all the time in physical problems, so you must be able to work with them confidently. Since a power of ten (the term 10^n) is part of every number written in scientific notation, the most important rules for dealing with such expressions are the Laws of Exponents:

Laws of Exponents		
		Illustration (with b = 10 or a power of 10)
Law 1	$b^p \times b^q = b^{p+q}$	$10^5 \times 10^{-9} = 10^{5+(-9)} = 10^{-4}$
Law 2	$b^p/b^q = b^{p-q}$	$10^5/10^{-9} = 10^{5-(-9)} = 10^{14}$
Law 3	$(b^p)^q = b^{pq}$	$(10^{-3})^2 = 10^{(-3)(2)} = 10^{-6}$
Law 4	$b^0 = 1$ (if $b \ne 0$)	$10^0 = 1$
Law 5	$b^{-p} = 1/b^p$	$10^{-7} = 1/10^7$
Law 6	$(ab)^p = a^p b^p$	$(2 \times 10^4)^3 = 2^3 \times (10^4)^3 = 8 \times 10^{12}$
Law 7	$(a/b)^p = a^p/b^p$	$[(3 \times 10^{-6})/10^2]^2 = (3 \times 10^{-6})^2/(10^2)^2 = 9 \times 10^{-16}$

Example 13-1: Simplify each of the following expressions, writing your answer in scientific notation:

a) $(4 \times 10^{-3})(5 \times 10^9)$
b) $(4 \times 10^{-3})/(5 \times 10^9)$
c) $(3 \times 10^{-4})^3$
d) $[(1 \times 10^{-2})/(5 \times 10^{-7})]^2$

Solution:

a) $(4 \times 10^{-3})(5 \times 10^9) = (4)(5) \times 10^{-3+9} = 20 \times 10^6 = 2 \times 10^7$
b) $(4 \times 10^{-3})/(5 \times 10^9) = (4/5) \times 10^{-3-9} = 0.8 \times 10^{-12} = 8 \times 10^{-13}$
c) $(3 \times 10^{-4})^3 = 3^3 \times (10^{-4})^3 = 27 \times 10^{-12} = 2.7 \times 10^{-11}$
d) $[(1 \times 10^{-2})/(5 \times 10^{-7})]^2 = (1 \times 10^{-2})^2/(5 \times 10^{-7})^2 = (1 \times 10^{-4})/(25 \times 10^{-14}) = (1/25) \times 10^{-4-(-14)}$
   $= (4/100) \times 10^{10} = 4 \times 10^8$

Another important skill involving numbers written in scientific notation involves changing the power of 10 (and compensating for this change so as not to affect the original number). The approximation carried out in the very first example in this chapter is a good example of this. To find the square root of 5×10^{-7}, it is much easier to first rewrite this number as 50×10^{-8}, because then the square root is easy:

$$\sqrt{50 \times 10^{-8}} = \sqrt{50} \times \sqrt{10^{-8}} \approx 7 \times 10^{-4}$$

Other examples of this procedure are found in Example 13-1 above; for instance,

$$20 \times 10^6 = 2 \times 10^7$$

$$0.8 \times 10^{-12} = 8 \times 10^{-13}$$

$$27 \times 10^{-12} = 2.7 \times 10^{-11}$$

In writing $\sqrt{50 \times 10^{-8}} = \sqrt{50} \times \sqrt{10^{-8}} \approx 7 \times 10^{-4}$, I used a familiar law of square roots, that the square root of a product is equal to the product of the square roots. Here's a short list of rules for dealing with radicals:

Laws of Radicals		
		Illustration
Law 1	$\sqrt{ab} = \sqrt{a} \cdot \sqrt{b}$	$\sqrt{9 \times 10^{12}} = \sqrt{9} \times \sqrt{10^{12}} = 3 \times 10^6$
Law 2	$\sqrt{a/b} = \sqrt{a}/\sqrt{b}$	$\sqrt{(4 \times 10^{-6})/10^{-18}} = \sqrt{(4 \times 10^{-6})}/\sqrt{10^{-18}} =$ $(2 \times 10^{-3})/10^{-9} = 2 \times 10^6$
Law 3	$\sqrt[q]{a^p} = a^{p/q}$	$\sqrt[3]{(8 \times 10^6)^2} = (8 \times 10^6)^{2/3} = 8^{2/3} \times 10^{(6)(2/3)} = 4 \times 10^4$

A couple of remarks about this list: First, Laws 1 and 2 illustrate how to handle square roots, which are the most common. However, the same laws are true even if the index of the root is not 2. [The **index** of a root (or radical) is the number that indicates the root that's to be taken; it's indicated by the little q in front of the radical sign in Law 3. Cube roots are index 3 and written $\sqrt[3]{\ }$; fourth roots are index 4 and written $\sqrt[4]{\ }$; and square roots are index 2 and written $\sqrt[2]{\ }$, although we hardly ever write the little 2.] Second, Law 3 provides the link between exponents and radicals.

Example 13-2: Approximate each of the following expressions, writing your answer in scientific notation:

a) $\sqrt{3.5 \times 10^9}$

b) $\sqrt{8 \times 10^{-11}}$

c) $\sqrt{\dfrac{1.5 \times 10^{-5}}{2.5 \times 10^{-17}}}$

Solution:

a) $\sqrt{3.5 \times 10^9} = \sqrt{35 \times 10^8} = \sqrt{35} \times \sqrt{10^8} \approx \sqrt{36} \times \sqrt{10^8} = 6 \times 10^4$

b) $\sqrt{8 \times 10^{-11}} = \sqrt{80 \times 10^{-12}} = \sqrt{80} \times \sqrt{10^{-12}} \approx \sqrt{81} \times \sqrt{10^{-12}} = 9 \times 10^{-6}$

c) $\sqrt{\dfrac{1.5 \times 10^{-5}}{2.5 \times 10^{-17}}} = \dfrac{\sqrt{1.5 \times 10^{-5}}}{\sqrt{2.5 \times 10^{-17}}} = \dfrac{\sqrt{15 \times 10^{-6}}}{\sqrt{25 \times 10^{-18}}} \approx \dfrac{\sqrt{16} \times \sqrt{10^{-6}}}{\sqrt{25} \times \sqrt{10^{-18}}} = \dfrac{4 \times 10^{-3}}{5 \times 10^{-9}} = 0.8 \times 10^6 = 8 \times 10^5$

Example 13-3: Approximate each of the following expressions, writing your answer in scientific notation:

a) The mass (in grams) of 4.7×10^{24} molecules of CCl_4:
$$\frac{(4.7 \times 10^{24})(153.8)}{6.02 \times 10^{23}}$$

b) The electrostatic force (in newtons) between the proton and electron in the ground state of hydrogen:
$$\frac{(8.99 \times 10^9)(1.6 \times 10^{-19})^2}{(5.3 \times 10^{-11})^2}$$

Solution:

a) $$\frac{(4.7 \times 10^{24})(153.8)}{6.02 \times 10^{23}} \approx \frac{5(150)}{6} \times 10^{24-23} = 5(25) \times 10 = 1.25 \times 10^3$$

b) $$\frac{(8.99 \times 10^9)(1.6 \times 10^{-19})^2}{(5.3 \times 10^{-11})^2} \approx \frac{9(1.6)^2 \times 10^{9+(-19)(2)}}{(5.3)^2 \times 10^{(-11)(2)}} \approx \frac{(9)3 \times 10^{-29}}{27 \times 10^{-22}} = 1 \times 10^{-7}$$

13.3 FRACTIONS, RATIOS, AND PERCENTS

A **fraction** indicates a division; for example, 3/4 means 3 divided by 4. The number above (or to the left of) the fraction bar is the numerator, and the number below (or to the right) of the fraction bar is called the denominator.

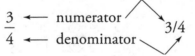

$$\frac{3}{4} \quad \begin{array}{l} \leftarrow \text{numerator} \\ \leftarrow \text{denominator} \end{array} \quad 3/4$$

Our quick review of the basic arithmetic operations on fractions begins with the simplest rule: the one for multiplication:

$$\frac{a}{b} \times \frac{c}{d} = \frac{ac}{bd}$$

In words, just multiply the numerators and then, separately, multiply the denominators.

Example 13-4: What is 4/9 times 2/5?

Solution:

$$\frac{4}{9} \times \frac{2}{5} = \frac{4 \times 2}{9 \times 5} = \frac{8}{45}$$

The rule for dividing fractions is based on the reciprocal. If $a \neq 0$, then the **reciprocal** of a/b is simply b/a; that is, to form the reciprocal of a fraction, just flip it over. For example, the reciprocal of 3/4 is 4/3; the reciprocal of –2/5 is –5/2; the reciprocal of 3 is 1/3; and the reciprocal of –1/4 is –4. (The number 0 has no reciprocal.) As a result of this definition, we have the following basic fact: The product of any number and its reciprocal is 1.

Example 13-5: Find the reciprocal of each of these numbers:

a)   2.25
b) 5×10^{-4}
c) 4×10^{5}

Solution:

a)   2.25 is equal to 2 + (1/4), which is 9/4. The reciprocal of 9/4 is 4/9.

b) $$\frac{1}{5 \times 10^{-4}} = \frac{1}{5} \times \frac{1}{10^{-4}} = 0.2 \times 10^{4} = 2 \times 10^{3}$$

c) $$\frac{1}{4 \times 10^{5}} = \frac{1}{4} \times \frac{1}{10^{5}} = 0.25 \times 10^{-5} = 2.5 \times 10^{-6}$$

Now, in words, the rule for dividing fractions reads: *multiply by the reciprocal of the divisor.* That is, flip over whatever you're dividing by, and then multiply:

$$\frac{a}{b} \div \frac{c}{d} = \frac{a}{b} \times \frac{d}{c}$$

Example 13-6: What is 4/9 divided by 2/5?

Solution:

$$\frac{4}{9} \div \frac{2}{5} = \frac{4}{9} \times \frac{5}{2} = \frac{4 \times 5}{9 \times 2} = \frac{20}{18} = \frac{10}{9}$$

Finally, we turn to addition and subtraction. In elementary and junior high school, you were probably taught to find a common denominator (preferably, the *least* common denominator, known as the LCD), rewrite each fraction in terms of this common denominator, then add or subtract the numerators. If a common denominator is easy to spot, this may well be the fastest way to add or subtract fractions:

$$\frac{1}{2} + \frac{3}{4} = \frac{2}{4} + \frac{3}{4} = \frac{2+3}{4} = \frac{5}{4}$$

However, it's now time to learn the grown-up way to add or subtract fractions:

$$\frac{a}{b} + \frac{c}{d} = \frac{ad + bc}{bd} \qquad\qquad \frac{a}{b} - \frac{c}{d} = \frac{ad - bc}{bd}$$

Here's what the arrows in the top line represent: "Multiply *up* (*d* times *a* gives *ad*), multiply *up* again (*b* times *c* gives *bc*), do the adding or subtracting of these products, and place the result over the product of the denominators (bd)." The length of this last sentence hides the simplicity of the rule, but it describes the recipe to follow. For example,

$$\frac{4}{9}+\frac{2}{5}=\frac{20+18}{45}=\frac{38}{45} \qquad \frac{4}{9}-\frac{2}{5}=\frac{20-18}{45}=\frac{2}{45}$$

Example 13-7:

a) Approximate the sum $\dfrac{1}{2.4\times10^5}+\dfrac{1}{6\times10^4}$

b) What is the reciprocal of this sum?

c) Simplify: $\dfrac{1}{2\times10^{-8}}-\dfrac{2}{5\times10^{-7}}$

Solution:

a) Using the rule illustrated above, we find that

$$\frac{1}{2.4\times10^5}+\frac{1}{6\times10^4}=\frac{(6\times10^4)+(2.4\times10^5)}{(2.4\times10^5)(6\times10^4)}=\frac{(6\times10^4)+(24\times10^4)}{(2.4\times10^5)(6\times10^4)}=\frac{(6+24)\times10^4}{(2.4)(6)\times10^{5+4}}\approx\frac{30\times10^4}{15\times10^9}=2\times10^{-5}$$

b) The reciprocal of this result is $\dfrac{1}{2\times10^{-5}}=\dfrac{1}{2}\times\dfrac{1}{10^{-5}}=0.5\times10^5=5\times10^4$.

c) $$\frac{1}{2\times10^{-8}}-\frac{2}{5\times10^{-7}}=\frac{(5\times10^{-7})-(2\times10^{-8})(2)}{(2\times10^{-8})(5\times10^{-7})}=\frac{(50\times10^{-8})-(4\times10^{-8})}{(2)(5)\times10^{-8+(-7)}}=\frac{(50-4)\times10^{-8}}{10\times10^{-15}}=46\times10^6$$
$$=4.6\times10^7$$

Let's now move on to ratios. A **ratio** is simply another way of saying *fraction*. For example, the ratio of 3 to 4, written 3:4, is equal to the fraction 3/4. Here's an illustration using isotopes of chlorine: The statement *the ratio of ^{35}Cl to ^{37}Cl is 3:1* means that there are 3/1 = 3 times as many ^{35}Cl atoms as there are ^{37}Cl atoms.

A particularly useful way to interpret a ratio is in terms of parts of a total. A ratio of $a:b$ means that there are $a + b$ total parts, with a of them being of the first type and b of the second type. Therefore, *the ratio of ^{35}Cl to ^{37}Cl is 3:1* means that if we could take all ^{35}Cl and ^{37}Cl atoms, we could partition all them into 3 + 1 = 4 equal parts such that 3 of these parts will all be ^{35}Cl atoms, and the remaining 1 part will all be ^{37}Cl atoms. We can now restate the original ratio as a ratio of these parts to the total. Since ^{35}Cl atoms account for 3 parts out of the 4 total, the ratio of ^{35}Cl atoms to all Cl atoms is 3:4; that is, 3/4 of all Cl atoms are ^{35}Cl atoms. Similarly, the ratio of ^{37}Cl atoms to all Cl atoms is 1:4, which means that 1/4 of all Cl atoms are ^{37}Cl atoms.

Example 13-8: The formula for the compound TNT (trinitrotoluene) is $C_7H_5N_3O_6$.

a) What fraction of the atoms in this compound are nitrogen atoms?
b) If the molar masses of C, H, N, and O are 12 g, 1 g, 14 g, and 16 g, respectively, what is the ratio of the mass of all the nitrogens to the total mass?

Solution:

a) There are a total of $7 + 5 + 3 + 6 = 21$ atoms per molecule. The ratio of N atoms to the total is 3:21, or, more simply, 1:7. Therefore, 1/7 of the atoms in this compound are nitrogen atoms.

b) The desired ratio of masses is calculated like this:

$$\frac{\text{mass of all N atoms}}{\text{total mass of molecule}} = \frac{3(14)}{7(12) + 5(1) + 3(14) + 6(16)} = \frac{42}{227} \approx \frac{40}{220} = \frac{2}{11}$$

Example 13-9: In a simple hydrocarbon (molecular formula C_xH_y), the ratio of C atoms to H atoms is 5:4, and the total number of atoms in the molecule is 18. Find x and y.

Solution: Since the ratio of C atoms to H atoms is 5:4, there are 5 parts C atoms and 4 parts H atoms, for a total of 9 equal parts. These 9 equal parts account for 18 total atoms, so each part must contain 2 atoms. Thus, C (which has 5 parts) has $5 \times 2 = 10$ atoms, and H (which has 4 parts) has $4 \times 2 = 8$ atoms. Therefore, $x = 10$ and $y = 8$.

Example 13-10: The ratio of O atoms to C atoms in each molecule of triethylene glycol is 2:3, and the ratio of O atoms to the total number of C atoms and H atoms is 1:5. If there are 24 atoms (C, H, and O only) per molecule, find the formula for this compound.

Solution: The ratio of O to C atoms is 2:3, which tells us there are 2 parts O atoms and 3 parts C atoms, for a total of 5 parts C and O. Since the ratio of O to (C *and* H) atoms is 1:5, there are 5 times as many C and H atoms as there are O atoms. But, we have found that there are 2 parts O atoms, so C and H must account for 5 times as many: 10 parts. And, because there are 3 parts C atoms, there must be $10 - 3 = 7$ parts H atoms. We therefore have $2 + 3 + 7 = 12$ parts total, accounting for 24 atoms, which means 2 atoms per part. So, there must be $2 \times 2 = 4$ O atoms, $3 \times 2 = 6$ C atoms, and $7 \times 2 = 14$ H atoms. The formula is $C_6H_{14}O_4$.

The word **percent**, symbolized by %, is simply an abbreviation for the phrase "out of 100". Therefore, a percentage is represented by a fraction whose denominator is 100. For example, 60% means 60/100, or 60 out of 100. The three main question types involving percents are as follows:

1) What is y % of z?
2) x is what percent of z?
3) x is y % of what?

Fortunately, all three question types fit into a single form and can all be answered by one equation. Translating the statement *x is y % of z* into an algebraic equation, we get

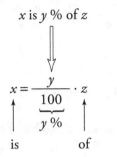

So, if you know any two of the three quantities *x*, *y*, and *z*, you can use the equation above to figure out the third.

Example 13-11:

a)   What is 25% of 200?
b)   30 is what percent of 150?
c)   400 is 80% of what?

Solution:

a)   Solving the equation $x = (25/100) \times 200$, we get $x = 25 \times 2 = 50$.
b)   Solving the equation $30 = (y/100) \times 150$, we get $y = (30/150) \times 100 = (1/5) \times 100 = 20$.
c)   Solving the equation $400 = (80/100) \times z$, we get $z = (100/80) \times 400 = 100 \times 5 = 500$.

It's also helpful to think of a simple fraction that equals a given percent, which can be used in place of $y/100$ in the equation above. For example, 25% = 1/4, 50% = 1/2, and 75% = 3/4. Other common fractional equivalents are: 20% = 1/5, 40% = 2/5, 60% = 3/5, and 80% = 4/5; 33 1/3% = 1/3 and 66 2/3% = 2/3; and 10n% = n/10 (for example, 10% = 1/10, 30% = 3/10, 70% = 7/10, and 90% = 9/10).

Example 13-12:

a)   What is 60% of 35?
b)   12 is 75% of what?
c)   What is 70% of 400?

Solution:

a)   Since 60% = 3/5, we find that $x = (3/5) \times 35 = 3 \times 7 = 21$.
b)   Because 75% = 3/4, we solve the equation $12 = (3/4) \times z$, and find $z = 12 \times (4/3) = 16$.
c)   Since 70% = 7/10, we find that $x = (7/10) \times 400 = 7 \times 40 = 280$.

Example 13-13:

a) What is the result when 50 is increased by 50%?
b) What is the result when 80 is decreased by 40%?

Solution:

a) "Increasing 50 by 50%" means adding (50% of 50) to 50. Since 50% of 50 is 25, increasing 50 by 50% gives us $50 + 25 = 75$.
b) "Decreasing 80 by 40%" means subtracting (40% of 80) from 80. Since 40% of 80 is 32, decreasing 80 by 40% gives us $80 - 32 = 48$.

Example 13-14:

a) What is 250% of 60?
b) 2400 is what percent of 500?

Solution:

a) Solving the equation $x = (250/100) \times 60$, we get $x = 25 \times 6 = 150$.
b) Solving the equation $2400 = (y/100) \times 500$, we get $2400 = 5y$, so $y = 2400/5 = 480$.

Example 13-15: There are three stable isotopes of magnesium: ^{24}Mg, ^{25}Mg, and ^{26}Mg. The relative abundance of ^{24}Mg is 79%. Consider a sample of natural magnesium containing a total of 8×10^{24} atoms.

a) About how many atoms in the sample are ^{24}Mg atoms?
b) If the number of ^{25}Mg atoms in the sample is 8×10^{23}, what is the relative abundance (as a percentage) of ^{25}Mg?
c) What's the relative abundance of ^{26}Mg?

Solution:

a) Since the question is asking, *What is 79% of 8×10^{24}?*, we have

$$x = \frac{79}{100} \times (8 \times 10^{24}) \approx \frac{80}{100} \times (8 \times 10^{24}) = 6.4 \times 10^{24}$$

b) The question is asking, *8×10^{23} is what percent of 8×10^{24}?*, so we write

$$8 \times 10^{23} = \frac{y}{100} \times (8 \times 10^{24}) \Rightarrow \frac{y}{100} = \frac{8 \times 10^{23}}{8 \times 10^{24}} = \frac{1}{10} \Rightarrow y = 10 \Rightarrow \text{relative abundance} = 10\%$$

c) Assuming that these three isotopes account for all naturally occurring magnesium, the sum of the relative abundance percentages should be 100%. Therefore, we need only solve the equation $79\% + 10\% + Y\% = 100\%$, from which we find that $Y = 11$.

Example 13-16: What is the percentage by mass of carbon in $C_7H_5N_3O_6$? (Given: Molar mass of compound = 227 g.)

A) 26%
B) 37%
C) 49%
D) 62%

Solution: Once the fraction of the total molar mass of the compound that's contributed by carbon is calculated, we obtain a percentage by multiplying this fraction by 100%. Since the molar mass of carbon is 12 g, and the molecule contains 7 C atoms, we have

$$\%C, \text{ by mass } = \frac{7(12)}{227} = \frac{84}{227} \approx \frac{100}{250} = \frac{2}{5} = \frac{2}{5} \times 100\% = 40\%$$

Therefore, choice B is best.

13.4 EQUATIONS AND INEQUALITIES

You may have several questions on the MCAT that require you to solve—or manipulate—an algebraic equation or inequality. Fortunately, these equations and inequalities won't be very complicated.

When manipulating an algebraic equation, there's basically only one rule to remember: *Whatever you do to one side of the equation, you must do to the other side.* (Otherwise, it won't be a valid equation anymore.) For example, if you add 5 to the *left*-hand side, then add 5 to the *right*-hand side; if you multiply the *left*-hand side by 2, then multiply the *right*-hand side by 2, and so forth.

Inequalities are a little more involved. While it's still true that whatever you do to one side of an inequality you must also do to the other side, there are a couple of additional rules, both of which involve flipping the inequality sign—that is, changing > to < (or vice versa) or changing ≥ to ≤ (or vice versa).

1) *If you multiply both sides of an inequality by a negative number, then you must flip the inequality sign.*

   For example, let's say you're given the inequality $-2x > 6$. To solve for x, you'd multiply both sides by $-1/2$. Since this is a negative number, the inequality sign must be flipped: $x < -3$.

2) *If both sides of an inequality are positive quantities, and you take the reciprocal of both sides, then you must flip the inequality sign.*

   For example, let's say you're given the inequality $2/x \leq 6$, where it's known that x must be positive. To solve for x, you can take the reciprocal of both sides. Upon doing so, the inequality sign must be flipped: $x/2 \geq 1/6$, so $x \geq 1/3$.

Example 13-17:

a) Solve for T: $PV = nRT$
b) Solve for v: $KE = (1/2)mv^2$
c) Solve for x (given that x is positive): $4x^2 = 2.4 \times 10^{-11}$
d) Solve for B: $h = k + \log(B/A)$
e) If $F = q_1q_2/r^2$ and r is positive, solve for r in terms of F, q_1, and q_2.
f) Solve for x: $3(2 - x) < 18$
g) Find all positive values of λ that satisfy

$$\frac{2 \times 10^{-25}}{\lambda} \geq 4 \times 10^{-19}$$

Solution:

a) Dividing both sides by nR, we get $T = PV/(nR)$.

b) Multiply both sides $2/m$, then take the square root: $v = \sqrt{\dfrac{2KE}{m}}$.

c) $4x^2 = 2.4 \times 10^{-11} \Rightarrow x^2 = 6 \times 10^{-12} \Rightarrow x = \sqrt{6} \times 10^{-6} \approx 2.5 \times 10^{-6}$

d) $h = k + \log\dfrac{B}{A} \Rightarrow \log\dfrac{B}{A} = h - k \Rightarrow 10^{h-k} = \dfrac{B}{A} \Rightarrow B = 10^{h-k} A$ [see Section 3.2]

e) $F = \dfrac{q_1q_2}{r^2} \Rightarrow r^2 = \dfrac{q_1q_2}{F} \Rightarrow r = \sqrt{\dfrac{q_1q_2}{F}}$

f) $3(2 - x) < 18 \Rightarrow 2 - x < 6 \Rightarrow -x < 4 \Rightarrow x > -4$

g) $\dfrac{2 \times 10^{-25}}{\lambda} \geq 4 \times 10^{-19} \Rightarrow \dfrac{\lambda}{2 \times 10^{-25}} \leq \dfrac{1}{4 \times 10^{-19}} \Rightarrow \lambda \leq \dfrac{2 \times 10^{-25}}{4 \times 10^{-19}} = 0.5 \times 10^{-6} \Rightarrow \lambda \leq 5 \times 10^{-7}$

13.5 THE *x-y* PLANE, LINES, AND OTHER GRAPHS

The figure below shows the familiar **x-y plane**, which we use to plot data and draw lines and curves showing how one quantity is related to another one:

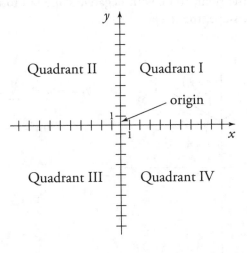

The *x-y* plane is formed by intersecting two number lines perpendicularly at the origins. The horizontal axis is generically referred to as the **x-axis** (although the quantity measured along this axis might be named by some other letter, such as time, *t*), and the vertical axis is generically known as the **y-axis**. The axes split the plane into four **quadrants**, which are numbered consecutively in a counterclockwise fashion. Quadrant I is in the upper right and represents all points (*x*, *y*) where *x* and *y* are both positive; in Quadrant II, *x* is negative and *y* is positive; in Quadrant III, *x* and *y* are both negative; and in Quadrant IV, *x* is positive and *y* is negative.

Suppose that two quantities, *x* and *y*, were related by the equation $y = 2x^2$. We would consider *x* as the **independent variable**, and *y* as the **dependent variable**, since for each value of *x* we get a unique value of *y* (that is, *y* *depends* uniquely on *x*). The independent variable is plotted along the horizontal axis, while the dependent variable is plotted along the vertical axis. Constructing a graph of an equation usually consists of plotting specific points (*x*, *y*) that satisfy the equation—in this case, examples include (0, 0), (1, 2), (2, 8), (−1, 2), (−2, 8), etc.—and then connecting these points with a line or other smooth curve. The first coordinate of each point—the *x* coordinate—is known as the **abscissa**, and the second coordinate of each point—the *y* coordinate—is known as the **ordinate**.

Lines

One of the simplest and most important graphs is the (straight) **line**. A line is determined by its slope—its steepness—and one specific point on the line, such as its intersection with either the *x*- or *y*-axis. The **slope** of a line is defined to be a change in *y* divided by the corresponding change in *x* ("rise over run"). Lines with positive slope rise to the right; those with negative slope fall to the right. And the greater the magnitude (absolute value) of the slope, the steeper the line.

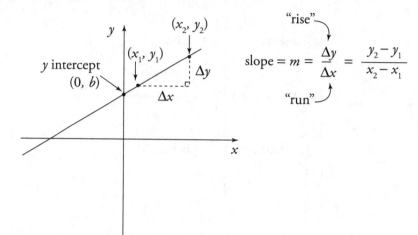

Perhaps the simplest way to write the equation of a line is in terms of its slope and the *y*-coordinate of the point where it crosses the *y*-axis. If the slope is *m* and the *y*-intercept is *b*, the equation of the line can be written in the form

$$y = mx + b$$

The only time this form doesn't work is when the line is vertical, since vertical lines have an undefined slope and such a line either never crosses the *y*-axis (no *b*) or else coincides with the *y*-axis. The equation of every vertical line is simply $x = a$, where *a* is the *x*-intercept.

Example 13-18:

a) Where does the line $y = 3x - 4$ cross the *y*-axis? the *x*-axis? What is its slope?
b) Find the equation of the line that has slope –2 and crosses the *y*-axis at the point (0, 3).
c) Find the equation of the line that has slope 4 and crosses the *y*-axis at the origin.
d) A *linear* function is a function whose graph is a line. Let's say it's known that some quantity *p* is a linear function of *x*. If $p = 50$ when $x = 0$ and $p = 250$ when $x = 20$, find an equation for *p* in terms of *x*. Then use the equation to find the value of *p* when $x = 40$.

Solution:

a) The equation $y = 3x - 4$ matches the form $y = mx + b$ with $m = 3$ and $b = -4$. Therefore, this line has slope 3 and crosses the *y*-axis at the point (0, –4). To find the *x*-intercept, we set *y* equal to 0 and solve for *x*: $0 = 3x - 4$ implies that $x = 4/3$. Therefore, this line crosses the *x*-axis at the point (4/3, 0).
b) We're given $m = -2$ and $b = 3$, so the equation of the line is $y = -2x + 3$.
c) We're given $m = 4$ and $b = 0$, so the equation of the line is $y = 4x$.
d) Since *p* is a linear function of *x*, it must have the form $p = mx + b$ for some values of *m* and *b*. Because $p = 50$ when $x = 0$, we know that $b = 50$, so $p = mx + 50$. Now, since $p = 250$ when $x = 20$, we have $250 = 20m + 50$, so $m = 10$. Thus, $p = 10x + 50$. Finally, plugging in $x = 40$ into this formula, we find that the value of *p* when $x = 40$ is $(10)(40) + 50 = 450$.

Example 13-19: An insulated 50 cm^3 sample of water has an initial temperature of $T_i = 10°C$. If Q calories of heat are added to the sample, the temperature of the water will rise to T, where $T = kQ + T_i$. When the graph of T vs. Q is sketched (with Q measured along the horizontal axis), it's found that the point $(Q, T) = (200, 14)$ lies on the graph.

a)   What is the value of k?
b)   How much heat is required to bring the water to 20°C?
c)   If $Q = 2200$ cal, what will be the value of T?

Solution:
a)   The equation $T = kQ + T_i$ matches the form $y = mx + b$, so k is the slope of the line. To find the slope, we evaluate the *rise-over-run* expression—which in this case is $\Delta T/\Delta Q$—for two points on the line. Using $(Q_1, T_1) = (0, 10)$ and $(Q_2, T_2) = (200, 14)$, we find that

$$k = \text{slope} = \frac{\Delta T}{\Delta Q} = \frac{T_2 - T_1}{Q_2 - Q_1} = \frac{14 - 10}{200 - 0} = \frac{1}{50}$$

b)   We set T equal to 20 and solve for Q:

$$T = kQ + T_i \Rightarrow T = \frac{1}{50}Q + 10 \Rightarrow 20 = \frac{1}{50}Q + 10 \Rightarrow Q = 500 \text{ (cal)}$$

c)   Here we set $Q = 2200$ and evaluate T:

$$T = kQ + T_i \Rightarrow T = \frac{1}{50}Q + 10 \Rightarrow T = \frac{1}{50}(2200) + 10 = 44 + 10 = 54 \text{ (°C)}$$

(*Technical note:* The equation for the temperature of the water, $T = kQ + T_i$, is valid as long as no phase change occurs.)

Besides lines, there are a few other graphs and features you should be familiar with.

The equation $y = kx^2$, where $k \neq 0$, describes the basic **parabola**, one whose turning point (**vertex**) is at the origin. It has a U shape, and opens upward if k is positive and downward if k is negative. The graph of the related equation $y = k(x - a)^2$ is obtained from the basic parabola by shifting it horizontally so that its vertex is at the point $(a, 0)$. The graph of the equation $y = kx^2 + b$ is obtained from the basic parabola by shifting it vertically so that its vertex is at the point $(0, b)$. Finally, the graph of the equation $y = k(x - a)^2 + b$ is obtained from the basic parabola in two shifting steps: First, shift the basic parabola horizontally so that its vertex is at the point $(a, 0)$; next, shift this parabola vertically so that the vertex is at the point (a, b). These parabolas are illustrated below for positive a, b, k, and x:

The equation $y = k/x$, where $k \neq 0$, describes a **hyperbola**. It is the graph of an inverse proportion (see Section 2.2). For small values of x, the values of y are large; and for large values of x, the values of y are small. Notice that the graph of a hyperbola approaches—but never touches—both the x- and y-axes. These lines are therefore called **asymptotes**.

The equation $y = k/x^2$, where $k \neq 0$, has a graph whose shape is similar to a hyperbola but it approaches its asymptotes faster than a hyperbola does (because of the square in the denominator).

The graph of the equation $y = Ae^{-kx}$ (where k is positive) is an **exponential decay curve**. It intersects the y axis at the point $(0, A)$, and, as x increases, the value of y decreases. Here, the x-axis is an asymptote.

The graph of the equation $y = A(1 - e^{-kx})$, where k is positive, contains the origin, and as x increases, the graph rises to approach the horizontal line $y = A$. This line is an asymptote.

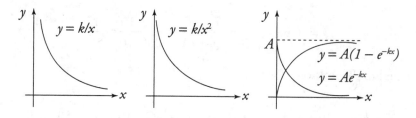

Chapter 14
Proportions

The concept of proportionality is fundamental to analyzing the behavior of many physical phenomena and is a common topic for MCAT questions.

14.1 DIRECT PROPORTIONS

If one quantity is always equal to a constant times another quantity, we say that the two quantities are **proportional** (or **directly proportional**, if emphasis is desired). For example, if k is some nonzero constant and the equation $A = kB$ is always true, then A and B are proportional, and k is called the **proportionality constant**. We express this fact mathematically by using this symbol: $\propto$, which means *is proportional to*. So, if $A = kB$, we'd write $A \propto B$. Of course, if $A = kB$, then $B = (1/k)A$, so we could also say that $B \propto A$.

Here are a few examples:

Example 14-1: Energy is equal to Planck's constant times frequency, $E = hf$. Therefore $E \propto f$.

Example 14-2: The ideal gas law states that $PV = nRT$. If n, V, and R are constant, $P \propto T$.

Example 14-3: The rate law for a chemical reaction that is first order with respect to reactant A is rate = k[A]. Assuming k is constant, rate $\propto$ [A].

The most important fact about direct proportions is this:

> *If $A \propto B$, and B is multiplied by a factor of b, then A will also be multiplied by a factor of b.*

After all, if $A = kB$, then $bA = k(bB)$.

Example 14-4: Since the energy of a photon is proportional to its frequency, $E \propto f$, then, if the frequency is doubled, so is the energy. If the frequency is reduced by half, so is the energy. If the frequency is tripled, so is the energy.

Example 14-5: Since the pressure inside a system is proportional to its temperature when volume and the number of moles present are constant, $P \propto T$, when the temperature is quadrupled, the pressure is quadrupled. When the pressure is decreased by a factor of 3, the temperature is also decreased by a factor of 3.

Example 14-6: Since the rate of a first order chemical reaction is proportional to the concentration of reactant A, [rate] $\propto$ [A], if [A] is increased by a factor of 2, the rate also increases by a factor of 2. If [A] is decreased by a factor of 4 (same as multiplying by ¼), the rate of reaction is ¼ of what it was originally.

It's important to notice that the actual numerical value of the proportionality constant was irrelevant in the statements made above. For example, the fact that h is the proportionality constant in the equation $E = hf$ did not affect the conclusions made above. If E and f were some other quantities and E happened to always be equal to (17,000)f, we'd still say $E \propto f$, and all the conclusions made in Example 14-4 above would still be correct.

Graphically, proportions are easy to spot. If the horizontal and vertical axes are labeled linearly (as they usually are), then *the graph of a proportion is a straight line through the origin*. Be careful not to make the common mistake of thinking that any straight line is the graph of a proportion. If the line doesn't go through the origin, then it's *not* the graph of a proportion.

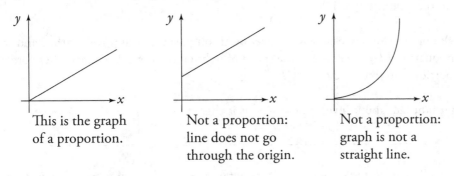

This is the graph of a proportion.

Not a proportion: line does not go through the origin.

Not a proportion: graph is not a straight line.

The examples we've seen so far have been the equations $E = hf$, $PV = nRT$, and *rate = k[A]*. Notice that in all of these equations, all the variables are present to the first power. But what about an equation like this: $KE = \frac{1}{2}mv^2$? This equation gives the kinetic energy of an object of mass m moving with speed v. So, if m is constant, KE is proportional to v^2. Now, what if v were multiplied by, say, a factor of 3, what would happen to KE? Because $KE \propto v^2$, if v increases by a factor of 3, then KE will increase by a factor of 3^2, which is 9. (By the way, this does not mean that if we graph KE versus v, we'll get a straight line through the origin. KE is not proportional to v; it's proportional to v^2. If we were to graph KE vs. v^2, *then* we'd get a straight line through the origin.) Here's another example using the same proportion, $KE \propto v^2$: If v were decreased by a factor of 2, then KE would decrease by a factor of $2^2 = 4$.

Here is one more example:

Example 14-7: The reaction quotient Q for a reaction is described by $Q = [A][B]^3$. Therefore, Q is proportional to the concentration of $[B]^3$: $Q \propto [B]^3$. So, for example, if $[B]$ were doubled, Q would increase by a factor $2^3 = 8$.

14.2 INVERSE PROPORTIONS

If one quantity is always equal to a nonzero constant *divided* by another quantity (that is, if $A = k/B$, where k is some constant), we say that the two quantities are **inversely proportional**. Here are two equivalent ways of saying this:

(i)   If the product of two quantities is a constant ($AB = k$), then the quantities are inversely proportional.

(ii) If A is proportional to $1/B$ [that is, if $A = k(1/B)$], then A and B are inversely proportional.

In fact, we'll use this final description to symbolize an inverse proportion. That is, if A is inversely proportional to B, then we'll write $A \propto 1/B$. (There's no commonly accepted single symbol for *inversely proportional to*.) Of course, if $A = k/B$, then $B = k/A$, so we could also say that $B \propto 1/A$.

Here are a couple of examples:

Example 14-8: The pressure P and volume V of a sample containing n moles of an ideal gas at a fixed temperature T is given by the equation $PV = nRT$, where R is a constant. Therefore, the pressure is inversely proportional to the volume: $P \propto 1/V$.

Example 14-9: For electromagnetic waves traveling through space, the wavelength λ and frequency f are related by the equation $\lambda f = c$, where c is the speed of light (a universal constant). Therefore, wavelength is inversely proportional to frequency: $\lambda \propto 1/f$.

The most important fact about inverse proportions is this:

> *If $A \propto 1/B$, and B is multiplied by a factor of b, then A will be multiplied by a factor of $1/b$.*

After all, if $A = k/B$, then $(1/b)A = k/(bB)$. Intuitively, if one quantity is *increased* by a factor of b, the other quantity will *decrease* by the same factor, and vice versa.

Example 14-10: Since the pressure of an ideal gas at constant temperature is inversely proportional to the volume, $P \propto 1/V$, then if the volume is doubled, the pressure is reduced by a factor of 2. If the volume is quadrupled, the pressure is reduced by a factor of 4. If the volume is divided by 3 (which is the same as saying it's multiplied by 1/3), then the pressure will increase by a factor of 3.

Example 14-11: Because for electromagnetic waves traveling through space, the wavelength is inversely proportional to frequency, $\lambda \propto 1/f$, if f is increased by a factor of 10, λ will decrease by a factor of 10. If the frequency is decreased by a factor of 2, the wavelength will increase by a factor of 2.

The graph of an inverse proportion is a *hyperbola*. In the graph below, $xy = k$, so x and y are inversely proportional to each other.

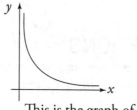

This is the graph of an inverse proportion.

The examples we've seen so far have been where one quantity is inversely proportional to the first power of another quantity. But what about an equation like this:

$$F = \frac{q_1 q_2}{r^2}$$

This equation gives the electrostatic force between two point charges of magnitude q_1 and q_2 separated by a distance r. So, if q_1 and q_2 are constant, F is inversely proportional to r^2. Now, if r were increased by, say, a factor of 3, what would happen to F? Because $F \propto 1/r^2$, if r increases by a factor of 3, then F will decrease by a factor of 3^2, which is 9. Here's another example using the same proportion, $F \propto 1/r^2$: If r were decreased by a factor of 2, then F would increase by a factor of $2^2 = 4$.

Example 14-12: Graham's law of effusion states that

$$\frac{\text{rate of effusion of Gas 1}}{\text{rate of effusion of Gas 2}} = \sqrt{\frac{m_2}{m_1}},$$

where m_2 is the molecular mass of Gas 2 and m_1 is the molecular mass of Gas 1. Therefore, the rate of effusion of Gas 1 is inversely proportional to the square root of its molecular mass, rate of effusion of Gas 1 $\propto \sqrt{\dfrac{1}{m_1}}$. So, if Gas 1 were changed to a molecule whose mass was 4 times greater, the rate of effusion of Gas 1 would decrease by a factor of 2.

Example 14-13: The kinetic energy of an object of mass m traveling with speed v is given by the formula $KE = mv^2/2$.
   a)   If v is increased by a factor of 6, what happens to KE?
   b)   In order to increase KE by a factor of 6, what must happen to v?

Solution:
   a)   Since $KE \propto v^2$, if v increases by a factor of 6, then KE increases by a factor of $6^2 = 36$.
   b)   Since $KE \propto v^2$, it follows that $\sqrt{KE} \propto v$. So, if KE is to increase by a factor of 6, then v must be increased by a factor of $\sqrt{6}$.

Chapter 15
Logarithms

15.1 THE DEFINITION OF A LOGARITHM

A **logarithm** (or just **log**, for short) is an exponent.

For example, in the equation $2^3 = 8$, 3 is the exponent, so 3 is the logarithm. More precisely, since 3 is the exponent that gives 8 when the base is 2,

$$\underset{\text{base}}{\overset{\text{exponent}}{\underset{\nearrow}{\overset{(\text{logarithm})}{\downarrow}}}} 2^3 = 8$$

we say that the base-2 log of 8 is 3, symbolized by the equation $\log_2 8 = 3$.

Here's another example: Since $10^2 = 100$, the base-10 log of 100 is 2; that is, $\log_{10} 100 = 2$. The logarithm of a number to a given base is the exponent the base needs to be raised to give the number. What's the log, base 3, of 81? It's the exponent we'd have to raise 3 to in order to give 81. Since $3^4 = 81$, the base-3 log of 81 is 4, which we write as $\log_3 81 = 4$.

The exponent equation $2^3 = 8$ is equivalent to the log equation $\log_2 8 = 3$; the exponent equation $10^2 = 100$ is equivalent to the log equation $\log_{10} 100 = 2$; and the exponent equation $3^4 = 81$ is equivalent to the log equation $\log_3 81 = 4$. For every exponent equation, $b^x = y$, there's a corresponding log equation: $\log_b y = x$, and vice versa. To help make the conversion, use the following mnemonic, called the *two arrows method*:

$$\log_2 8 = 3 \iff 2^3 = 8$$

$$\log_b y = x \iff b^x = y$$

You should read the log equations with the two arrows like this:

$$\log_2 \underset{\text{to the}}{8 = 3} \iff 2 \xrightarrow{\text{to the}} 3 \xrightarrow{\text{equals}} 8 \iff 2^3 = 8$$

$$\log_b \underset{\text{to the}}{y = x} \iff b \xrightarrow{\text{to the}} x \xrightarrow{\text{equals}} y \iff b^x = y$$

Always remember: The log is the exponent.

15.2 LAWS OF LOGARITHMS

There are only a few rules for dealing with logs that you'll need to know, and they follow directly from the rules for exponents (given earlier, in 13.2). After all, logs *are* exponents.

In stating these rules, we will assume that in an equation like $\log_b y = x$, the base b is a positive number that's different from 1, and that y is positive. (Why these restrictions? Well, if b is negative, then not every number has a log. For example, $\log_{-3} 9$ is 2, but what is $\log_{-3} 27$? If b were 0, then only 0 would have a log; and if b were 1, then every number x could equal $\log_1 y$ if $y = 1$, and *no* number x could equal $\log_1 y$ if $y \neq 1$. And why must y be positive? Because if b is a positive number, then b^x [which is y] is always positive, no matter what real value we use for x. Therefore, only positive numbers have logs.)

Laws of Logarithms	
Law 1	The log of a product is the sum of the logs: $\log_b (yz) = \log_b y + \log_b z$
Law 2	The log of a quotient is the difference of the logs: $\log_b (y/z) = \log_b y - \log_b z$
Law 3	The log of (a number to a power) is that power times the log of the number: $\log_b (y^z) = z \log_b y$

We could also add to this list that *the log of 1 is 0*, but this fact just follows from the definition of a log: Since $b^0 = 1$ for any allowed base b, we'll always have $\log_b 1 = 0$.

For the MCAT, the two most important bases are $b = 10$ and $b = e$. Base-10 logs are called **common** logs, and the "10" is often not written at all:

$$\log y \text{ means } \log_{10} y$$

The base-10 log is useful because we use a *decimal* number system, which is based (pun intended) on the number 10. For example, the number 273.15 means $(2 \times 10^2) + (7 \times 10^1) + (3 \times 10^0) + (1 \times 10^{-1}) + (5 \times 10^{-2})$. In physics, the formula for the decibel level of a sound uses the base-10 log. In chemistry, the base-10 log has many uses, such as finding values of the pH, pOH, pK_a, and pK_b.

Base-e logs are known as **natural** logs. Here, e is a particular constant, approximately equal to 2.7. This may seem like a strange number to choose as a base, but it makes calculus run smoothly—which is why it's called the *natural* logarithm—because (and you don't need to know this for the MCAT) the only numerical value of b for which the function $f(x) = b^x$ is its own derivative is $b = e = 2.71828\ldots$. Base-e logs are often used in the mathematical description of physical processes in which the rate of change of some quantity is proportional to the quantity itself; radioactive decay is a typical example. The notation "ln" (the abbreviation, in reverse, for **n**atural **l**ogarithm) is often used to mean $\log_e$:

$$\ln y \text{ means } \log_e y$$

The relationship between the base-10 log and the base-e log of a given number can be expressed as $\ln y \approx 2.3 \log y$. For example, if $y = 1000 = 10^3$, then $\ln 1000 \approx 2.3 \log 1000 = 2.3 \times 3 = 6.9$. You may also find it useful to know the following approximate values:

$$\log 2 \approx 0.3 \qquad \ln 2 \approx 0.7$$
$$\log 3 \approx 0.5 \qquad \ln 3 \approx 1.1$$
$$\log 5 \approx 0.7 \qquad \ln 5 \approx 1.6$$

Example 15-1:
a) What is $\log_3 9$?
b) Find $\log_5 (1/25)$.
c) Find $\log_4 8$.
d) What is the value of $\log_{16} 4$?
e) Given that $\log 5 \approx 0.7$, what's $\log 500$?
f) Given that $\log 2 \approx 0.3$, find $\log (2 \times 10^{-6})$.
g) Given that $\log 2 \approx 0.3$ and $\log 3 \times 0.5$, find $\log (6 \times 10^{23})$.

Solution:
a) $\log_3 9 = x$ is the same as $3^x = 9$, from which we see that $x = 2$. So, $\log_3 9 = 2$.
b) $\log_5 (1/25) = x$ is the same as $5^x = 1/25 = 1/5^2 = 5^{-2}$, so $x = -2$. Therefore, $\log_5 (1/25) = -2$.
c) $\log_4 8 = x$ is the same as $4^x = 8$. Since $4^x = (2^2)^x = 2^{2x}$ and $8 = 2^3$, the equation $4^x = 8$ is the same as $2^{2x} = 2^3$, so $2x = 3$, which gives $x = 3/2$. Therefore, $\log_4 8 = 3/2$.
d) $\log_{16} 4 = x$ is the same as $16^x = 4$. To find x, you might notice that the square root of 16 is 4, so $16^{1/2} = 4$, which means $\log_{16} 4 = 1/2$. Alternatively, we can write 16^x as $(4^2)^x = 4^{2x}$ and 4 as 4^1. Therefore, the equation $16^x = 4$ is the same as $4^{2x} = 4^1$, so $2x = 1$, which gives $x = 1/2$.
e) $\log 500 = \log (5 \times 100) = \log 5 + \log 100$, where we used Law 1 in the last step. Since $\log 100 = \log 10^2 = 2$, we find that $\log 500 \approx 0.7 + 2 = 2.7$.
f) $\log (2 \times 10^{-6}) = \log 2 + \log 10^{-6}$, by Law 1. Since $\log 10^{-6} = -6$, we find that $\log (2 \times 10^{-6}) \approx 0.3 + (-6) = -5.7$.
g) $\log (6 \times 10^{23}) = \log 2 + \log 3 + \log 10^{23}$, by Law 1. Since $\log 10^{23} = 23$, we find that $\log (6 \times 10^{23}) \approx 0.3 + 0.5 + 23 = 23.8$.

Example 15-2: In each case, find y.
a) $\log_2 y = 5$
b) $\log_2 y = -3$
c) $\log y = 4$
d) $\log y = 7.5$
e) $\log y = -2.5$
f) $\ln y = 3$

Solution:
a) $\log_2 y = 5$ is the same as $2^5 = y$, so $y = 32$.
b) $\log_2 y = -3$ is the same as $2^{-3} = y$, which gives $y = 1/2^3 = 1/8$.
c) $\log y = 4$ is the same as $10^4 = y$, so $y = 10,000$.
d) $\log y = 7.5$ is the same as $10^{7.5} = y$. We'll rewrite 7.5 as $7 + 0.5$, so $y = 10^{7+(0.5)} = 10^7 \times 10^{0.5}$. Because $10^{0.5} = 10^{1/2} = \sqrt{10}$, which is approximately 3, we find that $y \approx 10^7 \times 3 = 3 \times 10^7$.
e) $\log y = -2.5$ is the same as $10^{-2.5} = y$. We'll rewrite -2.5 as $-3 + 0.5$, so $y = 10^{-3+(0.5)} = 10^{-3} \times 10^{0.5}$. Because $10^{0.5} = 10^{1/2} = \sqrt{10}$, which is approximately 3, we have that $y \approx 10^{-3} \times 3 = 0.003$.
f) $\ln y = 3$ means $\log_e y = 3$; this is the same as $y = e^3$ (which is about 20).

Example 15-3: The definition of the pH of an aqueous solution is

$$pH = -\log [H_3O^+] \text{ (or, simply, } -\log [H^+])$$

where $[H_3O^+]$ is the hydronium ion concentration (in M).

Part I: Find the pH of each of the following solutions:
   a)   coffee, with $[H_3O^+] = 8 \times 10^{-6}\ M$
   b)   seawater, with $[H_3O^+] = 3 \times 10^{-9}\ M$
   c)   vinegar, with $[H_3O^+] = 1.3 \times 10^{-3}\ M$

Part II: Find $[H_3O^+]$ for each of the following pH values:
   d)   pH = 7
   e)   pH = 11.5
   f)   pH = 4.7

Solution:
   a) $pH = -\log(8 \times 10^{-6}) = -[\log 8 + \log(10^{-6})] = -\log 8 + 6$. We can now make a quick approximation by simply noticing that log 8 is a little less than log 10; that is, log 8 is a little less than 1. Let's say it's 0.9. Then $pH \approx -0.9 + 6 = 5.1$.
   b) $pH = -\log(3 \times 10^{-9}) = -[\log 3 + \log(10^{-9})] = -\log 3 + 9$. We now make a quick approximation by simply noticing that log 3 is about 0.5 (after all, $9^{0.5}$ *is* 3, so $10^{0.5}$ is close to 3). This gives $pH \approx -0.5 + 9 = 8.5$.
   c) $pH = -\log(1.3 \times 10^{-3}) = -[\log 1.3 + \log(10^{-3})] = -\log 1.3 + 3$. We can now make a quick approximation by simply noticing that log 1.3 is just a little more than log 1; that is, log 1.3 is a little more than 0. Let's say it's 0.1. This gives $pH \approx -0.1 + 3 = 2.9$.

Note 1:
We can generalize these three calculations as follows: If $[H_3O^+] = m \times 10^{-n}\ M$, where $1 \le m < 10$ and n is an integer, then the pH is between $(n - 1)$ and n; it's closer to $(n - 1)$ if $m > 3$ and it's closer to n if $m < 3$. (We use 3 as the cutoff since $\log 3 \approx 0.5$.)

---

   d)   If pH = 7, then $-\log[H_3O^+] = 7$, so $\log[H_3O^+] = -7$, which means $[H_3O^+] = 10^{-7}\ M$.
   e)   If pH = 11.5, then $-\log[H_3O^+] = 11.5$, so $\log[H_3O^+] = -11.5$, which means $[H_3O^+] = 10^{-11.5} = 10^{(0.5)-12} = 10^{0.5} \times 10^{-12} \approx 3 \times 10^{-12}\ M$.
   f)   If pH = 4.7, then $-\log[H_3O^+] = 4.7$, so $\log[H_3O^+] = -4.7$, which means $[H_3O^+] = 10^{-4.7} = 10^{(0.3)-5} = 10^{0.3} \times 10^{-5} \approx 2 \times 10^{-5}\ M$. $[10^{-0.3} \approx 2$ follows from the fact that $\log 2 \approx 0.3$.]

Note 2:
We can generalize these last two calculations as follows: If pH = $n.m$, where n is an integer and m is a digit from 1 to 9, then $[H_3O^+] = y \times 10^{-(n+1)}\ M$, where y is closer to 1 if $m > 3$ and closer to 10 if $m < 3$. (We take $y = 5$ if $m = 3$.)

Example 15-4: The definition of the pK_a of a weak acid is
$$pK_a = -\log K_a$$

where K_a is the acid's ionization constant.

15.2

Part I: Approximate the pK_a of each of the following acids:
a)   HBrO, with $K_a = 2 \times 10^{-9}$
b) HNO_2, with $K_a = 7 \times 10^{-4}$
c)   HCN, with $K_a = 6 \times 10^{-10}$

Part II: Approximate K_a for each of the following pK_a values:
d) $pK_a = 12.5$
e) $pK_a = 2.7$
f) $pK_a = 9.2$

Solution:

a) $pK_a = -\log (2 \times 10^{-9}) = -[\log 2 + \log (10^{-9})] = -\log 2 + 9$. We can now make a quick approximation by remembering that log 2 is about 0.3. Then $pK_a = -0.3 + 9 = 8.7$. Because the formula to find pK_a from K_a is exactly the same as the formula for finding pH from $[H^+]$, we could also make use of Note 1 in the solution to Example 15-3. If $K_a = m' \times 10^{-n}$ M, where $1 \le m < 10$ and n is an integer, then the pK_a is between $(n - 1)$ and n; it's closer to $(n - 1)$ if $m > 3$ and it's closer to n if $m < 3$. In this case, $m = 2$ and $n = 9$, so the pK_a is between $(n - 1) = 8$ and $n = 9$. And, since $2 < 3$, the pK_a will be closer to 9 (which is just what we found, since we got the value 8.7). Given a list of possible choices for the pK_a of this acid, just recognizing that it's a little less than 9 will be sufficient.

b)   With $K_a = 7 \times 10^{-4}$, we have $m = 7$ and $n = 4$. Therefore, the pK_a will be between $(n - 1) = 3$ and $n = 4$. Since $m = 7$ is greater than 3, the value of pK_a will be closer to 3 (around, say, 3.2).

c)   With $K_a = 6 \times 10^{-10}$, we have $m = 6$ and $n = 10$. Therefore, the pK_a will be between $(n - 1) = 9$ and $n = 10$. Since $m = 6$ is greater than 3, the value of pK_a will be closer to 9 (around, say, 9.2).

d)   If $pK_a = 12.5$, then $-\log K_a = 12.5$, so $\log K_a = -12.5$, which means $K_a = 10^{-12.5} = 10^{(0.5)-13} = 10^{0.5} \times 10^{-13} \approx 3 \times 10^{-13}$. We could also make use of Note 2 in the solution to Example 15-3. If $pK_a = n.m$, where n is an integer and m is a digit from 1 to 9, then $K_a = y \times 10^{-(n+1)}$ M, where y is closer to 1 if $m > 3$ and y is closer to 10 if $m < 3$. In this case, with $pK_a = 12.5$, we have $n = 12$ and $m = 5$, so the K_a value is $y \times 10^{-(12+1)} = y \times 10^{-13}$, with y closer to 1 (than to 10) since $m = 5$ is greater than 3 (this agrees with what we found, since we calculated that $K_a \approx 3 \times 10^{-13}$).

e)   With $pK_a = 2.7$, we have $n = 2$ and $m = 7$. Therefore, the K_a value is $y \times 10^{-(2+1)} = y \times 10^{-3}$, with y close to 1 since $m = 7$ is greater than 3. We can check this as follows: If $pK_a = 2.7$, then $-\log K_a = 2.7$, so $\log K_a = -2.7$, which means $K_a = 10^{-2.7} = 10^{(0.3)-3} = 10^{0.3} \times 10^{-3} \approx 2 \times 10^{-3}$.

f)   With $pK_a = 9.2$, we have $n = 9$ and $m = 2$. Therefore, the K_a value is $y \times 10^{-(9+1)} = y \times 10^{-10}$, with y closer to 10 (than to 1) since $m = 2$ is less than 3. We can say that $K_a \approx 6 \times 10^{-10}$.

Example 15-5:
a)   If y increases by a factor of 100, what happens to log y?
b)   If y decreases by a factor of 1000, what happens to log y?
c)   If y increases by a factor of 30,000, what happens to log y?
d)   If y is reduced by 99%, what happens to log y?

Solution:
a)   If y changes to $y' = 100y$, then the log increases by 2, since

$$\log y' = \log (100\, y) = \log 100 + \log y = \log 10^2 + \log y = 2 + \log y$$

b)   If y changes to $y' = y/1000$, then the log decreases by 3, since

$$\log y' = \log \left(\frac{y}{1000}\right) = \log y - \log 1000 = \log y - \log 10^3 = \log y - 3$$

c)   If y changes to $y' = 30{,}000y$, then the log increases by about 4.5, since

$$\log y' = \log (30000\, y) = \log 3 + \log 10000 + \log y \approx 0.5 + 4 + \log y = 4.5 + \log y$$

d)   If y is reduced by 99%, that means we're subtracting $0.99y$ from y, which leaves $0.01y = y/100$. Therefore, y has decreased by a factor of 100. And if y changes to $y' = y/100$, then the log decreases by 2, since

$$\log y' = \log \left(\frac{y}{100}\right) = \log y - \log 100 = \log y - \log 10^2 = \log y - 2$$

Example 15-6: A radioactive substance has a half-life of 70 hours. For each of the fractions below, figure out how many hours will elapse until the amount of substance remaining is equal to the given fraction of the original amount.
   a)   1/4
   b)   1/8
   c)   1/3

Solution:
   a)   After one half-life has elapsed, the amount remaining is 1/2 the original (by definition). After another half-life elapses, the amount remaining is now 1/2 of 1/2 the original amount, which is 1/4 the original amount. Therefore, a decrease to 1/4 the original amount requires 2 half-lives, which in this case is 2(70 hr) = 140 hr.
   b)   The fraction 1/8 is equal to 1/2 of 1/2 of 1/2; that is, $1/8 = (1/2)^3$. In terms of half-lives, a decrease to 1/8 the original amount requires 3 half-lives, which in this case is equal to 3(70 hr) = 210 hr. *In general, a decrease to $(1/2)^n$ the original amount requires n half-lives.*
   c)   The fraction 1/3 is not a whole-number power of 1/2, so we can't directly apply the fact given in the italicized sentence in the solution to part (b). However, 1/3 is between 1/2 and 1/4, so the time to get to 1/3 the original amount is between 1 and 2 half-lives. Since one half-life is 70 hr, the amount of time is between 70 and 140 hours; the middle of this range (since 1/3 is roughly in the middle between 1/2 and 1/4) is about 110 hours. The most general formula for calculating the elapsed time involves a logarithm: If $x < 1$ is the fraction of a radioactive substance remaining after a time t has elapsed, then

$$t = \frac{\log \frac{1}{x}}{\log 2} \times t_{1/2}$$

where $t_{1/2}$ is the half-life. (If you want to use this formula, remember that $\log 2 \approx 0.3$.)

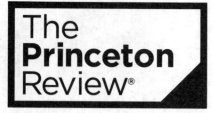

International Offices Listin

China (Beijing)
1501 Building A,
Disanji Creative Zone,
No.66 West Section of North 4th Ring Road Beijing
Tel: +86-10-62684481/2/3
Email: tprkor01@chol.com
Website: www.tprbeijing.com

China (Shanghai)
1010 Kaixuan Road
Building B, 5/F
Changning District, Shanghai, China 200052
Sara Beattie, Owner: Email: sbeattie@sarabeattie.com
Tel: +86-21-5108-2798
Fax: +86-21-6386-1039
Website: www.princetonreviewshanghai.com

Hong Kong
5th Floor, Yardley Commercial Building
1-6 Connaught Road West, Sheung Wan, Hong Kong
(MTR Exit C)
Sara Beattie, Owner: Email: sbeattie@sarabeattie.com
Tel: +852-2507-9380
Fax: +852-2827-4630
Website: www.princetonreviewhk.com

India (Mumbai)
Score Plus Academy
Office No.15, Fifth Floor
Manek Mahal 90
Veer Nariman Road
Next to Hotel Ambassador
Churchgate, Mumbai 400020
Maharashtra, India
Ritu Kalwani: Email: director@score-plus.com
Tel: + 91 22 22846801 / 39 / 41
Website: www.score-plus.com

India (New Delhi)
South Extension
K-16, Upper Ground Floor
South Extension Part–1,
New Delhi-110049
Aradhana Mahna: aradhana@manyagroup.com
Monisha Banerjee: monisha@manyagroup.com
Ruchi Tomar: ruchi.tomar@manyagroup.com
Rishi Josan: Rishi.josan@manyagroup.com
Vishal Goswamy: vishal.goswamy@manyagroup.com
Tel: +91-11-64501603/ 4, +91-11-65028379
Website: www.manyagroup.com

Lebanon
463 Bliss Street
AlFarra Building - 2nd floor
Ras Beirut
Beirut, Lebanon
Hassan Coudsi: Email: hassan.coudsi@review.com
Tel: +961-1-367-688
Website: www.princetonreviewlebanon.com

Korea
945-25 Young Shin Building
25 Daechi-Dong, Kangnam-gu
Seoul, Korea 135-280
Yong-Hoon Lee: Email: TPRKor01@chollian.net
In-Woo Kim: Email: iwkim@tpr.co.kr
Tel: + 82-2-554-7762
Fax: +82-2-453-9466
Website: www.tpr.co.kr

Kuwait
ScorePlus Learning Center
Salmiyah Block 3, Street 2 Building 14
Post Box: 559, Zip 1306, Safat, Kuwait
Email: infokuwait@score-plus.com
Tel: +965-25-75-48-02 / 8
Fax: +965-25-75-46-02
Website: www.scorepluseducation.com

Malaysia
Sara Beattie MDC Sdn Bhd
Suites 18E & 18F
18th Floor
Gurney Tower, Persiaran Gurney
Penang, Malaysia
Email: tprkl.my@sarabeattie.com
Sara Beattie, Owner: Email: sbeattie@sarabeattie.com
Tel: +604-2104 333
Fax: +604-2104 330
Website: www.princetonreviewKL.com

Mexico
TPR México
Guanajuato No. 242 Piso 1 Interior 1
Col. Roma Norte
México D.F., C.P.06700
registro@princetonreviewmexico.com
Tel: +52-55-5255-4495
+52-55-5255-4440
+52-55-5255-4442
Website: www.princetonreviewmexico.com

Qatar
Score Plus
Office No: 1A, Al Kuwari (Damas)
Building near Merweb Hotel, Al Saad
Post Box: 2408, Doha, Qatar
Email: infoqatar@score-plus.com
Tel: +974 44 36 8580, +974 526 5032
Fax: +974 44 13 1995
Website: www.scorepluseducation.com

Taiwan
The Princeton Review Taiwan
2F, 169 Zhong Xiao East Road, Section 4
Taipei, Taiwan 10690
Lisa Bartle (Owner): lbartle@princetonreview.com.tw
Tel: +886-2-2751-1293
Fax: +886-2-2776-3201
Website: www.PrincetonReview.com.tw

Thailand
The Princeton Review Thailand
Sathorn Nakorn Tower, 28th floor
100 North Sathorn Road
Bangkok, Thailand 10500
Thavida Bijayendrayodhin (Chairman)
Email: thavida@princetonreviewthailand.com
Mitsara Bijayendrayodhin (Managing Director)
Email: mitsara@princetonreviewthailand.com
Tel: +662-636-6770
Fax: +662-636-6776
Website: www.princetonreviewthailand.com

Turkey
Yeni Sülün Sokak No. 28
Levent, Istanbul, 34330, Turkey
Nuri Ozgur: nuri@tprturkey.com
Rona Ozgur: rona@tprturkey.com
Iren Ozgur: iren@tprturkey.com
Tel: +90-212-324-4747
Fax: +90-212-324-3347
Website: www.tprturkey.com

UAE
Emirates Score Plus
Office No: 506, Fifth Floor
Sultan Business Center
Near Lamcy Plaza, 21 Oud Metha Road
Post Box: 44098, Dubai
United Arab Emirates
Hukumat Kalwani: skoreplus@gmail.com
Ritu Kalwani: director@score-plus.com
Email: info@score-plus.com
Tel: +971-4-334-0004
Fax: +971-4-334-0222
Website: www.princetonreviewuae.com

Our International Partners

The Princeton Review also runs courses with a variety of partners in Africa, Asia, Europe, and South America.

Georgia
LEAF American-Georgian Education Center
www.leaf.ge

Mongolia
English Academy of Mongolia
www.nyescm.org

Nigeria
The Know Place
www.knowplace.com.ng

Panama
Academia Interamericana de Panama
http://aip.edu.pa/

Switzerland
Institut Le Rosey
http://www.rosey.ch/

All other inquiries, please email us at
internationalsupport@review.com